Handbook for Clinical
Investigators

Handbook for Clinical Investigators

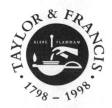

CHRISTOPHER T. KIRKPATRICK, BSc, MD, MFPM
Associate Director, Phase I Research
Chiltern International

TAYLOR & FRANCIS
ALERE FLAMMAM
·1798 – 1998·

UK   Taylor & Francis Ltd, 1 Gunpowder Square, London, EC4A 3DE
USA   Taylor & Francis Inc., 325 Chestnut Street, Philadelphia, PA 19106

British Library Cataloguing-in-Publication Data

A catalogue record for this book is available from the British Library.
ISBN 0-7484-0712-X (paper)

Library of Congress Cataloging-in-Publication Data are available

Cover design by Jim Wilkie
Typeset by Graphicraft Limited, Hong Kong
Printed and bound by T.J. International Ltd, Padstow, UK
Cover printed by Flexiprint, Lancing, West Sussex

Every effort has been made to ensure that the advice and information in this book is true and accurate at the time of going to press. However, neither the publisher nor the author can accept any legal responsibility or liability for any errors or omissions that may be made. In the case of drug administration, any medical procedure or the use of technical equipment mentioned within this book, you are strongly advised to consult the manufacturer's guidelines.

Contents

Preface

This book is aimed at potential clinical investigators, especially those thinking about doing clinical trials to evaluate new drugs. It is the attempt by one clinical investigator to share his experiences and insights, in the hope that others who might be attracted to the role of investigator can share in the excitement of clinical research while avoiding some of the pitfalls that inevitably beset the newcomer to clinical trials.

I have drawn upon my experiences as a research physician working first in a university, then in a government research institute, then in the mainstream pharmaceutical industry and a number of contract clinical research organisations. Most of my experience has been in the Phase I testing of drugs on healthy volunteers, but I have also seen a wide range of other types of interaction between sponsor and investigator, and between investigator and research subject (patient or volunteer). I believe I understand what the sponsor is looking for in a potential investigator, and also, how an investigator can get the best out of his sponsor!

Several books[1] are available which act as introductions to clinical research, and most contain sections relevant to the clinical investigator. They are largely distillations of the Good Clinical Practice guidelines as they apply to investigators, but are usually written from the point of view of the clinical trials manager or monitor. They try to explain the regulations to doctors in the hope of eliciting correct behaviour from them. I hope in this book to go beyond this, offering insights into what it means to be an investigator, and giving hints on how to survive in the jungle of Good Clinical Practice.

In some places in this book, persons fulfilling certain roles are referred to with either masculine or feminine pronouns. This is not to suggest that all investigators or doctors are men, or that all nurses or monitors are women, nor does it suggest that members of one or the other sex are better at fulfilling any particular role. It simply reflects the lack of a suitable neutral pronoun in English; it becomes tedious to keep saying him or her, (s)he or his/hers, so I have adopted the pronouns of the gender that comes most naturally to me. Most of the investigators I have met have been male (though I have met some very good female ones too) and most of the research nurses I have met have been female (though there are some very good male ones too). So please forgive any overt or covert gender bias in the text.

I owe a great deal to my present and former colleagues (who, with my past or present employers, must not be held responsible for any views expressed here – they are entirely my own). We have learnt a lot together, made some mistakes together (we have fortunately buried none of them!) and had a lot of fun together. I also owe a huge debt to the subjects (healthy volunteers or patients) who have participated in our trials, and have endured our ministrations with stoicism and even cheerful good humour. One of my volunteers, an American girl student, once said to me as I performed the screening examination for a trial: 'Gee, is it fun to be a physician?' and that put the whole enterprise into focus – clinical research is (or should be) fun.

CHRISTOPHER T. KIRKPATRICK

CHAPTER ONE

Motivation: What's in it for me?

By clinical research I mean the performance on human subjects of experimental procedures, trials and tests, usually of a therapeutic nature, with new drugs or new applications of older drugs. The term also encompasses the performance of purely physiological tests on humans, to find out either how drugs work or how humans work. A clinical investigator is someone who performs such experiments: he is usually a qualified physician or sometimes a dentist, or if he is scientifically qualified but has no specific medical training, he works very closely with a medical practitioner who provides 'medical cover'. Most drug regulatory authorities prefer their investigators to be medically qualified.

There are almost as many reasons for doing clinical research as there are investigators. Most of us do it with several simultaneous motives, sometimes conflicting or contradictory. Some do it because they have been asked to; others ask to do it. There are also many different career pathways to becoming a clinical investigator: some have undergone a recognised course of training for becoming an accredited clinical pharmacologist, or have spent years in the basic science or clinical laboratory, while others have come into research after years of experience in general practice or as a mainstream hospital clinician.

A clinical investigator may be an international authority on some important branch of therapeutics, or a member of a university department of pharmacology or medicine in a teaching hospital. Alternatively he may be a General Practitioner in his own surgery, a consultant or registrar in a District General Hospital or a physician in the purpose-built clinic of a major pharmaceutical company or a contract research organisation. Whatever his position, it is to be hoped that he has become an investigator primarily because he is interested in doing therapeutic research.

In the past, clinical research often proceeded in a piecemeal, *ad hoc* fashion as individual clinicians developed ideas and enthusiasms about possible therapeutic innovations, or drug companies found clinicians, sometimes on their own staff and sometimes in external institutions, to test their new products. People embarked on trials which were sometimes brilliant in conception, but were often of poor design and inadequate quality, so that drug development was a rather haphazard process. Nowadays clinical research is organised in a more formal planned manner, so that there is almost always a client/server or purchaser/provider relationship between a sponsor of research (such as a drug manufacturer or a research council) and the clinical investigator. The sponsor is responsible for checking that the investigator is performing the research according to the original concept and design, and according to internationally agreed standards of care and documentation. The investigator is responsible for recruiting patients or experimental subjects for the trial, and for their medical care while they are under study; he is also responsible for collecting the trial data according to the protocol or trial design.

The rules of evidence before a new product or procedure is accepted are more stringent and codified, and there is a risk that the excitement and flair associated with innovation in research could become submerged in a welter of detailed requirements for apparently trivial routine paperwork. Nevertheless the enthusiastic investigator must keep uppermost in his mind the original purpose of the trial, and try to maintain the sense of curiosity and inquiry which led him into clinical research in the first place.

1.1 HOW WE GOT THERE: APPROACH BY A SPONSOR

In one very common scenario, a sponsor company with a drug to be tested needs to find a team to perform the trial. The sponsor might wish to make use of the knowledge of a recognised expert in some particular field of medical science, to have a 'big name' associated with the project, and might invite him to become an investigator in the trial. Or the sponsor might approach several specialists in some clinical discipline to form a team of investigators for a multi-centre trial; this might be a given doctor's first experience of clinical research, but could represent an opportunity for him to enter the field, gaining experience and becoming an expert for subsequent trials.

A doctor might be attracted by an advertisement, or hear that a sponsor is seeking investigators for a trial, and might contact the sponsor, offering to take part. Some investigators may be drawn into research simply by being asked by a colleague to help; they find this first experience stimulating, and come back for more. Some potential investigators may be highly motivated to find a treatment or cure for a particular disease or condition, and will try to take part in any relevant trials that happen to be taking place in that field. Or an established and experienced practitioner working for a commercial contract research organisation might become involved because his company has just been awarded the contract to conduct the trial.

1.2 HOW WE GOT THERE:
APPROACH BY THE POTENTIAL INVESTIGATOR

In an alternative scenario a trial might be initiated by the investigator, rather than the sponsor. A medical scientist (either established or embryonic) might have an idea for an important piece of research, and might approach various sponsors including drug companies, charities or research funding councils for the necessary funds.[2] In such cases a grant application will be required, and each funding body will have its own forms of application and specify its own requirements for detailed proposals. The regulatory requirements for obtaining approval to proceed with the trial are also different for research initiated by investigators rather than pharmaceutical sponsors (in the UK a DDX is required – see the Glossary).

1.3 MISSION-DRIVEN OR CURIOSITY-DRIVEN RESEARCH

In projects initiated by individuals, or by groups in academic institutions or clinical practice, the main reasons for the research are usually scientific: this approach is often called curiosity-driven. (Other related motives include the desire for career advancement or for an increased number of publications.) If a drug company initiates the project, it is still quite possible for scientific questions to form a major part of the motivation, but almost every project will be conducted for a specific commercial reason, or for a regulatory purpose. These reasons may sometimes conflict with the scientific purpose. Such a project is referred to as mission-driven.

The balance between the scientific and the regulatory or commercial aspects may influence how interesting, attractive or publishable a project will be. There is a tendency to deprecate mission-driven research and to feel that curiosity-driven research is more 'pure' and therefore more praiseworthy; this is part of the snobbism of pure versus applied science, but in practice the distinction – probably artificial – between the two has become blurred;[3] most modern clinical research, whatever the motivation or the origin of the ideas, requires the participation of a large team of diverse individuals, not all of whom will have identical objectives, motives or roles.

1.4   REWARDS

Most investigators, once they have taken part in a research project, find it a very satisfying and rewarding activity (see the Preface: 'Gee, is it fun to be a physician?'). The thought of taking part in the development of an exciting new treatment, and the sense of belonging to a multi-disciplinary team achieving important goals can be stimulating. Lessons learnt about the discipline of scientific evaluation and the importance of recording everything can be transferred to other aspects of profes-sional life, and even in apparently mundane or routine projects the painstaking collection of accurate data can give a feeling of satisfaction.

1.4.1   Cash

Conducting clinical research can certainly augment the income of the investigator, and a few successful investigators manage to make a great deal of money out of it. The accusation is sometimes levelled that clinical investigators perform experiments on their patients for mercen-ary reasons – they prostitute their scientific ideals and may even com-promise patient safety for gain. I believe this is generally unfair and untrue – there are easier ways of making a lot of money – and most investigators are genuinely interested in the topic of the research. Even a physician in a contract research organisation (called upon to perform a wide variety of studies for a number of sponsors) does it because he is inherently interested in research – otherwise he would not be in the business.

For the majority of investigators, the income is not the primary or only motive, and most do not get particularly rich. Indeed, some inves-tigators plough all the income from their clinical trials back into their local research funds, or into a scientific travel fund for themselves or their staff. For many, especially in hospital units, the income from trials is used to fund the appointment of additional staff such as research nurses or research registrars, whose principal task is to help with the specific trial being funded, but who can also make a contribution to the department's overall clinical work and research effort in other projects.

1.4.2   Reputation and publication

Taking part in a successful clinical trial can add considerably to an investigator's scientific and clinical reputation, and may play an important part in getting promotion or professional advancement. The work may be published with the investigator as one of the authors, and this can contribute to the award of future research grants or to the investigator being asked to take part in future clinical trials. All of these, while being secondary motives, can contribute to the drive for an investigator to join the team for a particular trial.

1.5   THE MAIN TASK OF THE CLINICAL INVESTIGATOR

Whatever his own motivation, the investigator's primary role is to ensure the safety of his subjects or patients while they are in his care (see the preamble to the Declaration of Helsinki[4]). The search for financial or professional rewards or curiosity as to the outcome of the study must all be subservient to this role.

1.6   THE TEAM APPROACH

In almost all scientific research, and certainly in clinical research, the project depends upon a team rather than an individual scientist. The principal investigator in a clinical research project could well be a lone physician or other medical scientist, but more commonly is one among many. There will almost certainly also be clinicians at other sites, nurses, recruitment coordinators for patients or volunteers, data monitors, statisticians, pharmacists, finance officers and myriad other contributors to the overall success or failure of the project. The success of a research project depends, in large measure, on how successfully the team manages to work together, with each person making a valuable contribution to the whole, and each person deriving pride and satisfaction from the achievement of the whole. The clinical research investigator occupies, or should occupy, a key position in motivating and managing this team, but he too must be prepared to function as a member of the team rather than performing as a brilliant individualist. Part of the purpose of this book is to help the potential investigator navigate through the structure of the project team, and make use of the skills and abilities of the other team members as well as supporting them in making their contributions.

CHAPTER TWO

Brief overview of drug development

It takes about 12 years from first synthesis of a new molecule in the chemistry laboratory to the granting of marketing authorisation and the launch of a new drug. On average, six years are spent in basic pre-clinical research (chemistry, pharmacy, biology, pharmacology, toxicology) and a further six years in clinical development. Since the patent life of a newly-discovered molecule is 20 years, only a limited number of years is available for a drug manufacturer to make profits from marketing a successful new drug. After the patent expires, other companies are allowed to market generic copies without having to invest in the enormously expensive research and development programme which first brought the drug into clinical use. All pharmaceutical companies are therefore looking for ways to speed up the drug development process, and try to get the cooperation of everyone, including the clinical investigators, in making the process quick and smooth. Many companies, particularly the large ones, are now aiming to shorten the interval between molecular discovery and marketing authorisation to five or six years.

2.1 PRE-CLINICAL

The drug discovery process is often a mixture of serendipity (the chance finding of potentially useful molecules or naturally occurring products) and directed exploration. There is a trend in the mainstream pharmaceutical industry towards massive programmes for automated screening of new molecules, testing their ability to bind to a range of specific receptors; other approaches include computer-aided design of new drugs, based on a knowledge of the shape and properties of receptor sites or other drugs which are active at these sites. There is a huge investment in these screening programmes, but a very high attrition rate among the molecules: out of about 10,000 new molecules discovered in any year, only 100 may be of potential interest, only ten may reach clinical development and only one or two may reach the market. The process is very expensive: the price charged for a new drug has to reflect the cost of investigating all the failures as well as the cost of developing the successful drug.

Once a molecule has been identified as having potentially useful properties, a concerted effort goes into finding out all about its biological activity: how well and how selectively does it bind to its receptor, and what effect does it exert on cell fragments, the isolated cell, the isolated tissue or organ and the intact animal? The tasks of the biologist and the pharmacologist are to examine the potential beneficial effects of the drug and to predict how these might be useful in clinical practice. The real skill of the biologist is in devising models of human disease in animals or laboratory preparations: since many animals do not suffer from human diseases, we have to find some way to mimic the human condition in order to test a cure for it.

At the same time as the biological and pharmacological studies are proceeding, the drug is extensively examined by the toxicologist, to see what adverse effects there might be. Toxicology is the systematic study of possible harmful effects. It used to be common to perform a test called the LD_{50}, in which groups of animals were given progressively higher doses of the drug until half the animals in one group died (the Lethal Dose for 50 per cent). This test became the epitome of the anti-vivisectionist's case that research on animals was cruel and evil, and even among the research community the test was subject to a great deal of criticism, on the grounds that it was inhumane, gave information that was not directly relevant to the clinical use, and gave very little information about the toxic effects likely to be encountered in normal clinical use. The LD_{50} test has been replaced by a gentler and more gradual escalation of doses, trying to find the threshold at which sub-lethal toxic effects occur and recording the toxic effects much more carefully. The aim, before first giving the drug to humans, is to find the No Adverse Effect Level (NOAEL – or highest dose before toxicity occurs) on which to base the dosing schedule for the clinical studies.

The schedule of toxicity studies has become fairly standardised, beginning with acute or single-dose escalation studies, followed by subacute repeated dose studies lasting a few days, then chronic repeated dose studies. It is usual to delay single-dose studies in humans until the subacute toxicity has been studied in at least two animal species, and to defer any repeated dose studies in humans until the chronic toxicity (28 days) has been studied in two species (one of which should be non-rodent).

As well as simple toxicity, it is necessary to study the drug's capability to induce chromosomal changes or mutations (mutagenicity). This is usually studied *in vitro* in a number of systems, ranging from bacteria to fairly complex mammalian cell culture systems. If a drug fails the mutagenicity test it is very unlikely to be developed any further. It is also necessary to test for carcinogenicity: here the aim is to give a moderately high dose of a drug, but one that does not produce toxicity (and therefore cause the premature death of the animal), dosing the animal for the majority of its life-span. Any increase in the incidence of tumours or other malignant processes above the incidence found in control untreated or placebo-treated animals could indicate a potential for the drug to be carcinogenic to man, and usually leads to abandonment of the development programme for that drug.

There are also important studies to be done in reproductive toxicity, where the effects of the drug are studied on the ability of animals to conceive or to impregnate the female, on the ability to carry the fetus to term, and on the development of the fetus. A careful search is made for congenital abnormalities or deformities among the offspring (teratogenicity), as nobody wants a repetition of the Thalidomide tragedy where so many children were harmed by the drug taken by their mothers during pregnancy.[5]

Running in parallel with the biological and toxicity studies is the development of pharmaceutical formulation, looking for the most suitable way of delivering the drug to the target organ and producing a stable, convenient dosage form. The pharmaceutical development team also searches for the most efficient way of translating the chemical syntheses originally performed on a small scale in the test-tube into methods suitable for bulk production on an industrial scale.

There is often some overlap between the pre-clinical and clinical phases: the more long-term and expensive pre-clinical reproductive and teratogenicity studies are often delayed until after completion of the early human studies (using only male subjects, or females incapable of conception), to see whether or not the drug is in fact worth developing. Sometimes the findings in the early human studies can lead to new hypotheses which need to be tested in further animal experiments, or sometimes the product needs to be re-formulated in the light of clinical data.

2.2 CLINICAL

The clinical part of a drug's development usually consists of Phase I (the early trials on healthy volunteers to determine acute safety, pharmacokinetics, and perhaps some preliminary indications of efficacy); Phase II (the first trials in selected patients, where intensive studies are performed at specialist centres to measure key variables or indicators of disease in an attempt to verify the biological concepts and demonstrate efficacy); Phase III (extensive trials on large numbers of patients in a setting close to the intended clinical use of the drug, in general practice or the district general hospital) followed by submission of the regulatory dossier and (hopefully) licensing of the product; Phase IV (post-marketing surveillance for adverse effects, plus additional marketing support trials or exploration of new indications, new formulations, new combinations or interactions). Most of the pivotal studies of the clinical development programme, those that confirm the efficacy and safety of the drug in widespread use, are found in Phase III , and these are usually the studies to which the most resources are devoted.

2.3   DRUG REGISTRATION PROCEDURES

The procedures for obtaining a marketing licence for a new drug vary considerably from country to country, and it is important for the sponsor company to find out exactly what is required in the territory in which it intends to market the drug. Efforts are being made to afford mutual recognition among different licensing authorities, and it is now becoming the norm for companies in Europe developing new chemical entities to file their applications using the mutual recognition procedure. No matter where the application is being made, a dossier must be submitted to the drug licensing authorities containing details about all aspects of the drug's development: chemical synthesis, pharmaceutical formulation, biological and pharmacological activity, toxicology, and all the clinical trial data. The documents for a full submission to the licensing authority are very extensive, and can easily fill a small truck. The dossier contains all the original reports, summaries of the reports, and then summaries of the summaries.

CHAPTER THREE

Regulators and the Good Clinical Practice guidelines

3.1 THE GOOD CLINICAL PRACTICE DIRECTIVES

The agencies who give authorisation for marketing medicines in various regions (the European Union,[6] the US Food and Drug Administration[7] and now the International Committee on Harmonisation[8]) have issued guidelines or rules on how research on drugs should proceed: these define Good Clinical (Research) Practice (GCP). The guidelines describe the roles of the various parties involved in clinical research, including among others the sponsor (usually the drug manufacturer) and the investigator who conducts the research. Some of the investigator's functions are described in this chapter; the functions of the sponsor are described in the next. Despite differences in detail, the basic principles are the same. There are two main strands: protection of the research subject, and protection of the data.

3.1.1 Protection of the subject

The duty of the physician (and, by extension, any assistant to whom he delegates clinical tasks and duties) is primarily to his patient, to protect him from harm and if possible to treat his illness. During clinical research, the desire for scientific discovery or the impulse to reach a successful outcome must never be allowed to supersede this primary duty. The safety of the subject is the physician's chief responsibility, no matter what his job title, no matter who is paying him. The most important mechanisms for protection for the subject are: choice of competent investigators, review of all protocols by ethics committees, thorough monitoring by the sponsor's agent to ensure that the protocol and GCP guidelines are followed, and independent audit of safety issues.

3.1.2 Protection of the data

From the point of view of the regulators, the aim is to guard against fraud and the falsification or improper manipulation of data. From the point of view of the sponsor, the aim is to ensure good complete, correct, scientifically valid data on which sound conclusions and decisions can be based. From the investigator's point of view, it is unforgivable to expose volunteers or patients to risk in a trial in which the experimental question is poorly formulated, in which data are of poor quality or are ambiguously or inaccurately recorded, or in which records become lost or unusable.

From all points of view, it is desirable that the data be as complete and accurate as possible, and that as many pieces of information as possible be independently verifiable. Everything must be written down, preferably at the time the event occurs; unrecorded information may as well not exist. The main mechanisms to ensure integrity of the data are: thorough training of all research staff in correct and complete documentation; insistence on source document verification; checking of data by the investigator's staff, the sponsor's monitor, and the data management staff; and independent audit of all recording procedures and study documents.

3.1.3 European vs. USA requirements

There are differences in detail between the US FDA and the various European authorities over the interpretation of GCP and the documentary requirements, and each authority publishes extensive guidelines, rules and manuals. It is worth examining the main differences in culture and philosophy between US and European agencies: in general, the US authorities are *prescriptive* and the Europeans are *permissive* about what is to be done, what documents are to be submitted, and what rules are to be followed. Many of the FDA's officials regard themselves as *enforcement officers*. European officials are *assessors*. European agencies adopt the attitude: 'show us your dossier and we'll see whether we like it'. The European attitude is more flexible than that in the US, more susceptible to persuasion, more amenable to convincing by a well-reasoned argument, but on the other hand leaves greater scope for uncertainty. If one invests a great deal of time and effort, and succeeds in convincing the European agencies about an unconventional approach, the satisfaction is great. If one fails, the catastrophe and the disappointment are all the greater. With the US approach, one knows exactly where one stands – if all the prescribed trials are correctly completed, all the required documents are submitted and all the boxes on the forms are correctly ticked, the application will almost certainly be successful. On the other hand, there is little scope for the unusual, or for the unconventional approach.

With the coming of the International Committee on Harmonisation (ICH), these regional differences tend to disappear. Whilst standardisation and harmonisation are to be welcomed, the imposition of dull uniformity may take some of the flair and excitement out of clinical research. There is a growing tendency for monitors and auditors to insist on excessive documentation for documentation's sake, sometimes to the detriment of clinical care or the efficient performance of trial procedures, often provoking the investigator and his staff to lose sight of the scientific objective of the trial. There is therefore a need for responsible clinical investigators to stand up for themselves and for common sense, and be prepared to say 'don't be silly!'

3.2   ETHICAL ISSUES

3.2.1   Declaration of Helsinki

The Declaration of Helsinki (*Recommendations guiding physicians in biomedical research involving human subjects*) was issued by the World Medical Association after the end of the Second World War, when the horrors perpetrated in concentration camps were revealed, and the facts about human experimentation without consent became known. The Declaration has been subjected to periodic updates, the most recent in South Africa in 1996. Everyone quotes it, and attaches it to most protocols, but how many have read it in detail? I once saw a version which had been through a spell-check on the word processor, and every instance of 'subject' in the main protocol as well in the appendix containing the Declaration had been changed to 'patient'. It made a sort of sense most of the time, but there is a phrase about '. . . therapeutic value to the person *subjected* to the research . . .' where the spell-checker obviously suffered indigestion, and substituted 'patented' with no gain in clarity!

Despite all this, the Declaration is well worth reading, to bring us back to our fundamentals and constantly question what we are doing. The main message is that no point or principle, no form of scientific quest or curiosity can be more important than the safety and integrity of the human subject. The other important message is that, except in very special circumstances, all research subjects must be fully informed about the nature and risks of the trial and must give free, voluntary consent to take part.

3.2.2   Investigator

Probably the most important requirement for the conduct of ethical clinical trials is to have ethical investigators. The sponsors of trials must satisfy themselves absolutely that the investigators are well qualified practitioners of good standing, and are motivated to protect their patients and give them the best possible medical care. They must ensure that the investigators are thoroughly trained in the requirements of Good Clinical Practice and understand all the ethical implications of enrolling a subject in a clinical trial. They must be convinced that the investigators are honest and unlikely to generate fraudulent data.

3.2.3   Protocol design

One of the best means of protecting research subjects is the construction of a good protocol. It must be written with a view to patient safety from the outset, with careful checks built in to every stage of the design and with an emphasis on care and safety at every point in the execution of the trial. The safeguards of confidentiality and the requirements to obtain informed consent must be spelt out.

3.2.4   Ethics committee

All protocols, whether sponsored by the pharmaceutical industry, originating with the investigator or forming part of a project created by an academic unit or a research council, have to be approved by an independent ethics committee.

Many health boards or trusts in the UK NHS have set up Local Research Ethics Committees (LRECs), and there are even some regional Multi-centre Research Ethics Committees (MRECs). There is a feeling that these are the 'official' ethics committees, and that somehow the decisions made by other groups carry less weight and authority or might even be illegal. However, there is nothing in the Declaration of Helsinki, in law or in the GCP guidelines to say that an investigator has to consult the official LREC before embarking on a clinical trial (particularly on healthy volunteers); he is simply required to submit his protocol to an independent ethics committee. If he plans to use any National Health Service resources, then he is obliged by his NHS contract to consult the LREC constituted by the NHS, but this is an NHS regulation rather than the law, and many private ethics committees function very effectively, giving just as good protection to the research subjects as do the NHS committees. The private ethics committees usually act on protocols submitted by pharmaceutical companies or CROs, mainly for studies on healthy volunteers in their Phase I Units. They have often been in existence for much longer than the corresponding NHS committees, and consequently have a wealth of valuable experience which should not be ignored.

In other countries there are different regulations governing the exact composition and constitution of ethics committees (Institutional Review Boards in the US), but the principles remain the same: before any research proceeds on human subjects, there must be a written protocol describing the procedures, and it must be approved by an independent ethics committee. Most authorities now require that this approval be given in writing.

A properly constituted ethics committee should have specialist doctors and lay members, people of both sexes, members from the nursing profession and from General Practice, and preferably experts on relevant disciplines such as toxicology, statistics and the law. There may be representatives of minority ethnic groups, there may be clergy, or there may be representatives of health boards. The committee must be truly independent of the investigator, and able to call upon any specialist advice which cannot be supplied by its own members. It needs to have its own written standard procedures, to keep accurate minutes and to deal with its correspondence in a thoroughly professional way.

It is important to develop a good relationship with the Local Research Ethics Committee if you are going to do a significant amount of clinical research. Find out the local requirements for documents (number of copies of the protocol, any summary forms which they like, and document deadlines), but also try to get a feel for how the committee works, and what the members look for in assessing a project. If possible, have an informal meeting with the chairman or other key members, preferably over lunch – this should not be construed as trying to exert undue influence, but simply trying to find out what motivates the committee, and reassuring the committee of your *bona fides* as an investigator. Be prepared to attend meetings of the committee in order to explain details of the protocol – some committees like this, some insist on it, while others rarely ask investigators to attend except in unusual circumstances.

3.2.5   Temptations in an investigator's life

An investigator might be tempted, on initial approach by a sponsor's project leader or monitor looking for suitable investigator sites, *to inflate his ability to recruit subjects*. He should guard against entering into a contract to recruit unrealistic numbers of subjects, and against agreeing to unrealistic time-lines for recruitment, because serious failure to reach targets will detract from the overall success of the trial, and may well lead to the sponsor's excluding him from consideration as an investigator in future trials.

The temptation may exist *to squeeze subjects into the trial who may not be entirely appropriate*. This temptation must be resisted: first because the entry criteria for the trial are (or should be) designed to protect the subjects by preventing recruitment of persons for whom the trial might be dangerous, and second because a vigilant monitor is likely to spot any violation of the entry criteria, and will declare the subject unevaluable; the investigator will not get paid anyway. Even the honest investigator, entering subjects in good faith, will have to work hard to convince monitors that all his subjects meet the protocol requirements and are evaluable (and therefore attract a fee).

It is unfortunate that payment to investigators is almost always based on a head count; this could encourage a tendency to recruit inappropriately. The Royal College of Physicians' guidelines[9] suggested that this ought not to be the case, but realistically there is usually no other suitable basis on which to calculate payments. Even if fees were based on time rather than numbers of patients, the recruitment of inappropriate subjects could help to swell the apparent work-load to result in an inflated investigator grant. Do not lose sight of the primary responsibility: you are ultimately responsible for the patients' safety.

To conceal mistakes. Errors will inevitably occur. The automatic tendency is to try to conceal them, but this is likely to be counterproductive because of the intense scrutiny to which all aspects of clinical research are now subjected. A vigilant monitor or auditor is almost certain to notice discrepancies in recorded data and investigate further, leading to loss of credibility for the investigator, with the wrath of the sponsor who will vow never to use you as an investigator again; the sponsor may even withhold part or all of the investigator grant. It is better to be completely honest and inform the monitor as soon as you are aware of a mistake occurring; you are much more likely to elicit a sympathetic response than if you try to cover up. Coping strategies are discussed in a later section (Chapter 5).

To inflate the apparent efficacy. In a misguided attempt to please the sponsor, or in a vain attempt to substantiate your own pet hypothesis, you may be tempted to ascribe higher (or lower) scores than you actually find to key variables in your study, hoping to show that the treatment is efficacious. This is obviously a self-defeating strategy in double-blind projects, where you might be inflating the efficacy of the placebo treatment or your competitor's drug, but there are enough open trials around whose outcome could be influenced by a few manipulated numbers. Once again, a vigilant monitor may detect discrepancies, or a shrewd statistician may find values that fall outside the general trend and investigate the source of these spurious results. It is never worthwhile to record anything except the true data; even if you get away with deception, someone trying in the future to reproduce your results may find it impossible to do so, and cast doubts on the veracity of your study. It is also very irresponsible to falsify data that might lead to a drug being licensed when it is not actually as safe and efficacious as might appear.

Currently a high level of attention is given by the media to the subject of fraud in research, with entire issues of the *British Medical Journal*[10] being devoted to the problem, and watchdogs being set up by the authorities to guard against research fraud. It is a great pity that the topic is receiving so much adverse attention, as most researchers are still honest and simply want to get on with doing a good job, but the few high-profile fraudsters who have been caught have muddied the waters for the rest of us. Some regulatory authorities and auditors are now starting from the premise that every clinical investigator is a rogue and a fraud unless proved otherwise, and every document, every sample and every observation is being minutely scrutinised in an attempt to detect the dishonest entry which will invalidate an entire clinical trials programme.

3.3   THE DUTIES OF AN INVESTIGATOR

The duties and functions of investigators are usually self-evident and predictable using common sense, but they have now become codified by the various regulatory authorities and are listed in detail and at length in the various guideline documents. A brief overview of the main provisions is given here.

The investigator has a duty (which seems fairly obvious) to be thoroughly familiar with the use of the investigational product or experimental drug, and with the requirements of the protocol. He is expected to sign and agree with the protocol, and to submit it for scrutiny by an independent ethics committee before performing any study-related procedures. Once it is approved, he will follow the protocol without deviation, and without making up procedures, exceptions and additions as he goes along. He must ensure that all subjects entering the study have given informed consent, and must select only those subjects who meet the criteria specified in the protocol.

He is responsible for the medical care of his subjects, and for the behaviour and competence of any assistants whom he employs. He must ensure that adequate resources such as time, space and staff are available to conduct the trial properly and safely, and that all assistants receive thorough training both in the details of the protocol and in the methods of medical research.

He has a duty to take care of the investigational product, keeping supplies secure and maintaining adequate accountability. He has to keep accurate records of all clinical procedures and fill in the case report forms correctly; he has a duty to report all adverse events to the sponsor and to report serious adverse events immediately.

He is required to make available all study-related documents for scrutiny by the sponsor's monitors and auditors, and inspectors from the regulatory authority. This includes the case report forms, the subjects' original clinical notes, the investigator site file and any relevant correspondence.

3.3.1 The principal investigator

In many projects one of the investigators is designated as principal investigator, who has particular roles and responsibilities. Part of his role may be to act as one of the investigators in the trial, sometimes (as in small Phase I trials) the only one. He is expected to make a substantial contribution in an advisory capacity to project planning and protocol design. The principal investigator will often be chosen precisely because of his considerable experience and expertise in the scientific field of the trial, and will have valuable insights into methods, epidemiology and recruitment, and many practical aspects of study design. He will have a feel for what is feasible and what is unrealistic in a clinical setting. He may therefore be part of the group planning and writing the protocol, and should certainly be one of those who review it; he would be expected to sign the file copy of the protocol. He will be expected to give leadership to the other investigators in the trial, and might for example be one of the main speakers at the investigators' meeting.

Responsibility for the project

Like all other investigators, the principal investigator has a responsibility for the safety of his patients, but unlike the other investigators, this responsibility is not confined to the patients at his own centre: the principal investigator has an overall responsibility for all the subjects in the trial, and is often consulted over issues which impinge on safety of subjects in general rather than of particular subjects. The principal investigator will also take an overall view of the outcome of the study, and will often have access to and review the safety and efficacy data at a much earlier stage than the other investigators.

CTX responsibility

In trials conducted under a Clinical Trials Certificate Exemption (CTX) the principal investigator is often (but not always) the signatory of the CTX application, which makes him responsible for the accuracy of the data submitted to the Medicines Control Agency and gives him a duty to inform the MCA of any changes in the protocol and of any serious adverse events occurring during the trial.

3.4   THE CLINICAL TRIAL SUBJECT

3.4.1   The doctor–patient relationship is preserved

In any trial, the well-being of the subject is the physician's primary concern. You may be very interested in the scientific outcome of the trial, or at the more mundane level you may be keen to get your allotted quota of subjects enrolled for the trial in order to maximise your investigator grant, but such considerations must never be allowed to compromise the safety or rights of the individual subject. At all times, the essential doctor–patient relationship, which is built on trust and confidence, must be preserved. If you are a family physician or a hospital specialist recruiting your 'own' patients for the trial, a relationship of trust ought already to exist, and you must be careful not to abuse or exploit it unfairly. If you are an investigator who recruits subjects from the population at large, be aware that each of your recruits is some other doctor's patient, and you owe a duty, both to the patient and to the physician, to communicate effectively with the subject's family physician. You must also be at pains to develop a relationship of trust with the subject yourself, so that he or she feels confident in your explanation of the trial's aims and requirements, and is satisfied that the trial will result in no unpleasant surprises. The subject is entrusting you with the care of his or her health and future, and this is an awesome responsibility.

3.4.2   Informed consent

The basis of the Declaration of Helsinki is that participants in clinical trials must give informed consent. The giving of consent has three components: the provision to the subject of clear written information on the trial; the interview between the subject and investigator in which explanations are given and questions are asked and answered; and the consent form which is signed by the subject signifying that an adequate explanation has been given and that the subject gives his voluntary agreement to take part, while recognising his right to withdraw without prejudice at any time.

The information sheet

The sponsor often supplies a suggested subject information sheet as part of the protocol, and occasionally this will suffice to explain the trial to the potential subject. On the other hand, the supplied document is often written in such a turgid, technical style as to be totally incomprehensible to the average subject; this is particularly true of some documents originating from sponsors in the US. One of the ethics committees with which I have been associated insisted that all subject information sheets be written in such a way as to be intelligible to the average reader of one of the popular tabloid newspapers, and this is the standard of simplicity and clarity (if not the literary style) to which we must aspire. If the sponsor's supplied document fails to meet this criterion, then demand that it be re-drafted by the sponsor, or re-draft it yourself.

You must be perfectly happy about the information sheet which your subjects will read. Does it clearly lay out why the trial is being done? How the drug works? What is expected of the subject in terms of attendance, taking medication, undergoing test procedures or having blood samples collected? The hazards and inconveniences associated with the trial medication or procedures? How to get in touch if anything goes wrong? The possible advantages to the subject (including any honorarium or expenses payments)? No matter who drafts it, the subject information sheet is one of the documents that must be submitted to the ethics committee for its approval.

The consent form

The consent form may be attached to the information sheet, or may be a separate document. It, too, must be clear and comprehensible by the subjects. It must lay out what is being agreed, and to what treatment or procedures the consent is being given. If you are unhappy with the draft originally supplied by the sponsor, insist on a re-draft.

The recruiting interview

The initial interview with the prospective subject is a most important meeting. It is essential to handle it carefully and correctly to ensure on the one hand that the subject is fully aware of all the implications and expectations of being in the trial, but on the other hand that a potentially useful subject is not lost. It is worth spending time on this interview, to make sure you get things right. It is not the sort of thing that ought to be delegated to junior staff. The ICH GCP guidelines suggest that nurses or other assistants might be empowered to elicit consent for studies, but the interviewer, whoever he is, must always be someone who is thoroughly familiar with all aspects of the trial and who can accurately answer any questions that may arise. In most cases it should still be the physician who elicits consent.

Information is one important aspect; persuasion without undue pressure is another. If the patient or volunteer has the least doubt about the safety or discomfort of the trial, it would be wise not to keep trying to recruit him. A thorough check that the subject meets the entry criteria is essential, as there is nothing more disappointing or dispiriting for all concerned than to enrol a subject who subsequently has to be withdrawn because an eligibility criterion has been infringed. If there is the slightest doubt about a particular criterion, ask the monitor: a dispensation or waiver can sometimes be granted over minor deviations from the strict criteria, but only if it is sought in advance of starting the trial, and permission for such deviations must always be confirmed in writing.

3.5   STANDARD OPERATING PROCEDURES

The Good Clinical Practice directives state that sponsors must have procedural documents to define and describe in writing how all aspects of clinical research are to be conducted. These standard operating procedures (SOPs) must be followed during the execution of the research, and there are to be independent checks that they are being followed; this is one of the chief functions of the audit.

The possession of SOPs (and compliance with them) is mandatory for sponsors, but is also highly desirable for anyone else doing clinical research: essential for CROs, but also very useful for any investigational site. If you do not already have a set of SOPs, it may be well worth your while to write some. This not only impresses the monitors sent along by potential sponsors, but also makes it perfectly clear to your staff and colleagues what is expected of them when confronting subjects for clinical trials, or the documents or drugs.

3.5.1   The sponsor's SOPs

All sponsors will have sets of SOPs governing all the various types of interaction with investigators, and often describing how investigators should behave. There will be SOPs (complete with extensive checklists) on investigator selection, on how to conduct placement visits, initiation visits, routine monitoring visits, close-down visits, and even how to answer the telephone. They expect these to be followed – don't be alarmed, they are usually very helpful in focusing the mind on the problem, and will repay careful study, providing suggestions on how you might frame your own set of SOPs.

3.5.2   The contract research organisation's SOPs

All contract research organisations will have a set of SOPs to cover the various activities involved in clinical research, or else will implement and enforce the SOPs of the sponsor company for the duration of the trial. You are well advised to find out from the CRO whose SOPs are to be followed, and to read those which are relevant to your participation in the trial, so that you know what to expect. Compare the SOPs of the sponsor or CRO with your own (see below), to find out whether there is any conflict between the requirements of one set of SOPs and another. There should be very little scope for conflict in these days of harmonisation, since if each set of SOPs is constructed according to the ICH guidelines, they will end up looking very similar.

3.5.3 Your own SOPs (you should have some!)

If you are serious about becoming involved in clinical research, give some concentrated thought to creating a set of SOPs for your own site or department. The writing of SOPs requires only some skill but a lot of common sense – they need to be clearly written and easy to follow and they must describe the functions accurately. If they are too complex or unreasonably demanding, they get ignored or are not properly followed: they then become no more than decorations on the walls or shelves of the clinical research department or your own office. Look at someone else's SOPs as an example (either of how to do it or how not to do it), or ask a CRA or monitor to help you to draft some. Don't try to be too clever: simply describe step by step how to perform each task.

3.5.4 Compliance

Writing SOPs is only the first step: you next have to follow them or enforce them. The best way to have them followed is to write them clearly and simply, make all your staff aware of their existence, explain the need for having them, and emphasise the need for compliance. Regular training is essential, and staff must be asked to sign a document, usually kept with the training records, stating that they have read and understood the relevant SOPs and intend to comply with them. Monitors and auditors will want to see your SOPs, and will want to know what you are doing to ensure compliance.

CHAPTER FOUR

The sponsor

4.1 THE PROJECT TEAM

For each new drug in development, the sponsor company creates a project team to decide what studies need to be performed and who should do them, and then to oversee the progress of the studies. Some very senior scientists, physicians, statisticians and project planners might be involved in the team, but the person who will interact most closely with the investigator is the monitor.

A typical clinical project team might consist of a project manager, usually a senior CRA (scientist) but occasionally a senior physician; several CRAs who act as study monitors; one or more medical advisers who advise on medical aspects of protocol development, oversee issues of subject safety and contribute to the safety analysis during the reporting stage; statisticians who ideally contribute at an early stage to protocol design, supervise the randomisation or other allocation of treatments, and conduct the statistical analysis of the study data at the time of reporting; data managers who are responsible for gathering the data written in the case report forms, ensuring their correctness and completeness, and translating them into an electronic database ready for the statistician. There may also be a variety of pharmacists to arrange packing, labelling and distribution of clinical trials supplies, document clerks to coordinate the shipping of study materials and documents to and from the investigators, and coordinators of laboratory investigations. A clinical trial can be a very complex operation indeed.

4.2   THE MONITOR

The monitor is the main contact between the sponsor and the investigator. In most companies the monitor or clinical research associate (CRA) has a life science degree (often a higher degree such as a PhD), but in some instances a CRA may be a physician or dentist, a nurse or a pharmacist. Whatever the background, the monitor ought to have undergone intensive in-job and external training in the requirements, methods and organisation of clinical trials, and should represent a most valuable resource to any investigator.

Although the monitor is an employee of the sponsor, and acts as the agent of the sponsor, the clever investigator should be able to make good use of the monitor to get all sorts of help and ensure the smooth running of the project. The primary task of the monitor is to ensure on behalf of the sponsor that the project runs to time, smoothly and correctly according to the protocol, so anything that the investigator may need to facilitate execution of the trial can come within the CRA's remit.

Look upon the CRA as your friend, as a resource rather than a nuisance or the annoying agent of the sponsor who is always checking up on you. For example, if you need access to particular references or documents, the monitor may well be able to track them down, using the resources of the sponsor company. If you need a particular type of form to be designed and produced to help you organise things or gather data, ask the monitor rather than trying to do it yourself. In some cases a monitor may be able to help you get essential items of equipment, perhaps on loan or on hire, such as a small centrifuge or even a computer.

The monitor will spend a lot of time checking things: before the trial, the facilities for conducting the investigation, for storing the drugs, for keeping the paperwork, the correspondence with ethics committees, the investigator's *curriculum vitae*; during the trial, the inventory of drugs and the dispensing records, the completion of the case report forms, the correct filing of documents, the progress of patient recruitment, the storage and shipping of blood and urine samples; after the trial the filling in of all sorts of forms, the resolution of data queries, the collection of unused medication, the follow-up of any adverse events or abnormalities in pathology laboratory tests.

It is the job of the monitor to check everything, and this has to be done for every investigator, so do not get irritated if queries are raised or mistakes are pointed out: it does not imply personal criticism of you as an investigator, and it happens to everyone. If CRAs go home in the evening without having found some problem to resolve, they do not get 'the gratifying feeling that our duty has been done' (W.S. Gilbert, *The Gondoliers*). The trick is to try to keep the number of queries to a minimum – you can play a game with the CRA, anticipating the queries and trying to circumvent them, but you will not win! Maintain a light and good-humoured relationship with the CRA, and try to enlist him or her as an ally, getting as much help out of the sponsor as possible.

4.2.1 Source document verification

The monitor has a duty to verify information in the CRF against independent source documents, wherever possible. It is thus essential that source documents be made available to the monitor (or auditor). They may not take away copies, but are required to check that the documents (and the patients) exist, and that they support the information entered in the CRF. Details such as the subject's identity, sex, date of birth, medical history and particularly details concerning diagnosis of the condition pertinent to the trial will always need to be confirmed, as will visit dates and the obtaining of informed consent, as well as any adverse events. Suitable source documents are items such as patient notes, laboratory reports, x-rays and ECG reports. I shall deal in a later section (Chapter 5) with the keeping of notes, but all of the usual kinds of clinical records can act as source documents.

4.3 AUDIT

All clinical research is now supposed to be subject to independent audit: that is a third party (the auditor), independent both of the sponsor's clinical project team and of the investigator, is to be allowed access to the facilities and documents of the research project, in order to verify and certify that all requirements of Good Clinical Practice are being satisfied and that the protocol is being correctly followed. Auditors should be treated with the same courtesy as the CRAs from the sponsor company, and their function is not to trap the unwary investigator or engage in punitive rebuke; they are there, as are most of the members of the research community, to help fulfil the basic requirements of GCP: protection of the subjects, and protection of the data.

There will be times when auditors or monitors, in their zeal to be seen to conform with their own visions of Good Clinical Practice, will make demands, suggestions or requests that are bizarre, odd, downright annoying, clearly outrageous or just plain daft. Investigators must not hesitate in such circumstances, to say 'Don't be silly!' There is a need for investigators to be prepared to stand up to the sillier exponents of GCP, to defend their own actions and justify their practices, both on grounds of common sense and in keeping with the original aims and objectives of GCP. Auditors and monitors making suggestions perceived as silly by the investigator must likewise be prepared to justify their demands by pointing out the section of the GCP guidelines that demands the particular odd activity.

4.4　THE CONTRACT

Every investigator embarking on a clinical trial for a sponsor will be given a contract describing what is expected from each party and what each party expects in return. Make certain you have an agreed and signed contract before you start, otherwise you may run into all sorts of difficulties in the middle of the trial, and if things are not written down the solution is hard to find. The contract might be directly between the investigator and the sponsor, or there may be a contract with the CRO who in turn has a contract with the sponsor.

4.4.1　Financial details

Make sure that all important details are taken care of, and be very firm in insisting that the whole contract is to your satisfaction. It is almost certainly worth showing it to your financial or legal adviser. Be sure that you have agreed on how much money is to be paid, and for what services. On what basis is the investigator grant to be calculated? At what milestones are payments to be made? Which currency is to be used? At what exchange rate? Is payment to be made with or without deduction of tax? Is Value Added Tax involved? Into whose bank account is it to be paid? What penalties are there in the contract on either side, to allow for things like late supply of trial medication on the part of the sponsor or failure of recruitment on the part of the investigator?

Are you being paid a fair fee for the work involved? Talk to colleagues who have been involved in clinical research to get a feel for what is a suitable level for an investigator grant, and what clauses in the contracts are reasonable or unreasonable; compare the fees to the recommended scales for private medical work published by your local medical association. Check the timing of staged payments, and beware the contract that pays the fee only on receipt of properly completed case report forms; a great deal of time can be spent in performing relatively minor corrections, and meanwhile your money is sitting in the sponsor's bank! Even worse is the contract that specifies payment only on receipt of the final report, as reports can take years rather than months to finalise, by the time they have been seen, modified and approved by all the relevant levels of management.

Look carefully to see whether the institution in which you are working (university or hospital) has put in a claim for overheads in addition to the investigator grant. It is becoming the norm for the host institution to claim anything from 10 per cent to 50 per cent in addition to the investigator fee for the use of the premises and facilities. Do you think it is fair? Is the institution going to contribute to the research project by the amount of the claimed overheads? Will its claim for these overheads deter your sponsor from using you again in the future?

Are 'pass-through' costs to be paid by the sponsor? For example, will the sponsor pay for laboratory tests, in particular for any extra follow-up tests if someone develops an abnormality? Who pays for subjects who fail screening, who withdraw because of adverse experiences, or who withdraw for other (including social) reasons? Are funds available to allow patients to be brought to your premises by taxi, or are mileage payments available? Be insistent that you (and your subjects) are not to be left with extra out-of-pocket expenses, and do not allow the clinical trial to leave you worse off financially than if you had not taken part.

Are funds available to pay a fee to the subjects? It is customary to offer a fee to healthy volunteers in Phase I trials, but in my view all subjects in clinical trials deserve to be paid for their time, and the inconvenience involved in taking part. This should not be looked on as an inducement, but as a recognition of the subject's contribution to the success of the project. Admittedly a patient in a therapeutic trial might derive some direct clinical benefit from taking part, but who derives the greatest benefit? It is almost certainly the sponsor, who completes the trial and soon gets the product to market. The investigator also benefits; he gets his fee, a fillip to his scientific reputation and his publication record, and the gratitude of the sponsor. The patient may wish selflessly to contribute to medical knowledge about his condition, but is likely to gain only transient benefit himself for the duration of the trial, after which he must return to his older established treatment or no treatment; he runs the risk of having no treatment at all in a placebo-controlled trial; he is subjected to a barrage of extra tests, procedures and investigations, additional visits, restrictions on diet or lifestyle, or the requirement to keep a diary of symptoms and medication. He deserves to have some reward for his valuable contribution to scientific and medical progress.

4.4.2 What the sponsor will provide

The sponsor must provide a protocol, an investigator brochure, case report forms and supplies of study medication. Make sure you know whether any additional supplies are to be provided, such as specimen bottles and labels, special equipment such as centrifuges, or additional stationery.

Ensure that you know what insurance cover or indemnity is provided. The sponsor of trials in the UK should agree to abide by the ABPI guidelines on compensation, either for clinical trials or for non-patient volunteer trials (the provisions are slightly different, and rather more generous for volunteer trials). These mean that if a subject suffers injury as a result of receiving experimental medication (or in the case of a volunteer, as a result of being in the trial) compensation will be available without the subject's having to prove negligence in court (no-fault compensation). Most contracts stipulate that compensation is only payable if the protocol was being correctly followed, so it is important for the investigator to make sure his own membership of a medical protection organisation is up to date and to check just what that membership covers, as sometimes there are special restrictions or special subscription rates for clinical trials.

4.4.3 What the investigator will provide

The investigator is contracted to find patients or subjects to take part in the study procedures, and collect data for the case report forms. He is contracted to provide clinical supervision or care for the subjects, and to report any adverse experiences to the sponsor. He is obliged to allow access to documents and notes to the sponsor's monitor or auditor, and inspectors from national regulatory bodies; this permits them to verify the accuracy of the data in the CRFs and ensure that the trial was conducted correctly in accordance with the protocol, the SOPs and the provisions of the relevant GCP guidelines.

4.4.4 Confidentiality

Patient data

The patient clinical notes at your hospital, health centre or clinic are always confidential documents, and the names, addresses and other identifying features must never be published or communicated to the sponsor. The sponsor's monitor or auditor, who also have a duty of confidentiality, may be allowed to see the patient notes and lists of names or dates of birth for purposes of verification, but must not take them away or make copies. The monitor and auditor have a duty to check that informed consent has been given, and so must be allowed to see the signed documents, but should not normally take away copies (an exception must be made for French sponsors, since French law requires that the sponsor retain copies of consent forms in a sealed envelope, only to be opened in exceptional circumstances such as a lawsuit arising from a clinical trial). Always remember the provisions of the Data Protection Act[11] in cases where personally identifiable information about subjects is kept on a computer: the subject must be informed that computer records exist, must be given a copy of the information if requested, and may request correction or deletion of the details.

All data on CRFs must be anonymised: the subject is given a trial identifier (such as a randomisation number) which is entered on all the CRF pages, and the only other identifiers are the subject's initials and date of birth. Any correspondence with the sponsor about an individual subject must quote the subject number rather than the name, and any supporting documents attached to the CRF such as laboratory reports or ECG traces should also be anonymised. Naturally the monitor is bound by the same rules of confidentiality as all of the clinical staff, and must not divulge to a third party any personal information seen during the scrutiny of patient or volunteer records.

Problems can arise where the employees of a pharmaceutical company act as volunteers in the company's Phase I unit, and their records might be seen by colleagues in the company. I have seen an instance where the clinical research nurse also acted as the occupational health nurse for the company, and the screening examinations for the trials were performed in the same place and by the same staff as the pre-employment examinations. There is obviously considerable scope for conflict of interest here, as health problems divulged to trials staff might affect the subject's employability. For instance, a positive test for drugs of abuse or for human immunodeficiency virus (HIV) might have serious consequences if the employer found out.

Product data

An investigator will have access to data regarding the drug and its development which may be commercially sensitive. He must not divulge any details of the drug's properties or the sponsor's development plan to anyone outside the project, nor must he use the knowledge so gained to buy and sell stocks or shares in the company at an advantage over others who do not have access to this information (this is insider trading and is illegal as well as unethical).

Trial data

The fact that a trial is taking place, and details of the protocol, results of clinical efficacy tests or the rate of recruitment and drop-out of subjects might be of value to a competitor or might even affect a company's value on the stock exchange, and must be kept secret. Investigators have a duty to maintain confidentiality about the progress and results of a trial, until the sponsor in discussion with the investigators has decided that the time is ripe to publish the results. In a later section I discuss the investigator's duty to publish if he feels that information which ought to be public is being suppressed, but before any steps are taken in this direction there must be full discussions with the sponsor – such action must not be taken lightly or in secret.

4.5   THE PROTOCOL

The protocol represents your map or guide through the project. It should contain detailed instructions on how to perform all procedures at each stage of the study, what to do at each visit, how to cope with problems and how to record the data.

During the planning phase you must insist on reviewing the protocol before it is finalised; beware the sponsor who comes to you with an already complete protocol and a 'take it or leave it' attitude. You should scrutinise the draft protocol very thoroughly, to make sure it contains all the things you want to see. It will usually have been produced by people thoroughly familiar with Good Clinical Practice, but you should check the following: Does it adequately reflect the scientific background? Are the aims clearly stated? Does it allow us to achieve the aims? Does it properly describe how to collect the data required? Are any important details left out? Could the average scientifically trained reader execute the procedures accurately by following the instructions? Do

you and your staff fully understand everything contained in the protocol? Do you feel ethically, scientifically and clinically comfortable
about all the things the protocol requires? Is it feasible in the specified
time-frame and with the given resources?

If you find anything in the draft with which you disagree, or which
you do not understand, tell the sponsor immediately and insist that it
be changed. As the investigator, you are the person responsible for
implementing the protocol, so make sure that you have a document
which you feel is workable. If the sponsor won't change, talk to the
principal investigator and see if he can bring pressure to bear; if you
still don't get satisfaction, you can always decline to take part, and must
hold true to your principles and beliefs.

Make sure that the section on compensation for study-related or
drug-related injury is satisfactory. There are differences in the compensation available for non-therapeutic and therapeutic trials; there are
marked differences between the cover offered to subjects or patients
in the United States and Europe. Insist that the level of cover provided
is appropriate: for example in the UK the sponsor should (as a minimum) follow the most recent ABPI guidelines,[12] and there must be a
statement in the protocol to that effect. The sponsor should provide
'no-fault' compensation (not just payment of medical·expenses, as is
common in US trials) for any trial-related injury (not only injury by the
sponsor's drug, but also injury experienced while receiving placebo
or comparator treatment, or while undergoing trial-related procedures.
For example, a subject might faint during venepuncture and suffer
head injury – not a drug-related injury but clearly a trial-related injury).
Ask for sight of the sponsor's insurance policy if possible.

Once you have accepted and agreed the protocol, you must go
through it in detail, preferably with the study site coordinator, and
translate it into practice: in other words, work out exactly what must
be done, at what time and in what sequence, at each visit. Look at the
draft CRF, and see whether it corresponds with the protocol, allowing
you to capture the data in a simple logical and unambiguous way. If
you detect deficiencies in the CRF, or if you can foresee snags in how
the data are to be recorded, then draw up a worksheet or time-table for
your own use, which directs the collection of the data in a way that
you and your team find convenient. The careful translation of the protocol into action is a most important step in your participation in the
trial.

Become thoroughly familiar with the protocol, and if necessary con-
struct working summaries or copy extracts for ready reference. For
example, you may find it convenient to keep a copy of the admission

criteria beside you while you are screening potential subjects. It may be useful to pin copies of the flow-chart or schedule on the walls of the study room, or in the sleeping or eating quarters of the subjects so that they know when they are expected to have a blood sample taken or have a measurement of blood pressure.

4.6   STRUCTURE

The typical protocol will contain the following information (though not necessarily in this order or format: companies vary widely in their SOPs about protocol writing, though all the contents should be broadly similar).

4.6.1   Introduction

A statement about the target disease, and the scientific background to the drug about to be tested. Any information available about previous human trials, especially about safety issues. The objectives of the trial must be clearly stated.

4.6.2   Subject population

A full description of the eligibility criteria. Look at these very closely, for they often determine the feasibility or otherwise of the study. Look in particular at the allowed concomitant or previous medication, and the statements about pre-existing conditions.

4.6.3   Description of test articles (i.e. drugs)

A full description of how the study medication is to be formulated, packed, supplied and labelled. Full information must also be available about placebo or comparator medication.

4.6.4   Procedures and methods

This is the most important section of any protocol, and must contain a detailed description of all procedures at each visit, with instructions on actions to be taken if things go wrong or problems occur.

4.6.5 Statistical and analytical methods

There must be a full description of how the data are to be processed and analysed, together with a justification for the sample size to be used. Do not be satisfied with protocols which essentially say (usually clothed in considerable jargon) 'we will make up the analytical plan as we go along, once we see the data'.

There should also be a description of the laboratory analytical methods to be used, for example in pharmacokinetic trials or in trials involving unusual or non-routine laboratory investigations. Do not allow the sponsor to get away with statements like 'samples will be shipped to the laboratory for analysis of plasma concentrations'. We need to know at least which technique (such as HPLC, RIA or ELISA) is to be used, and what is the limit of detection or quantification. We need to be assured that the technique is actually capable of measuring the drug in the samples which we collect, otherwise we are wasting our time!

4.6.6 Ethical and GCP issues

The protocol must contain details of how ethics committee approval is to be sought, how informed consent is to be elicited from the subjects, and how the subjects' rights and safety are to be safeguarded (this includes information on compensation of subjects). It must also contain details of how monitors and auditors are to be allowed access to data, and instructions on the correct collection of clinical data and the making of changes or corrections.

4.6.7 Administrative issues

Matters such as contact addresses and telephone numbers, how to report serious adverse events, and the proposed start and finish dates of the study should be mentioned. Make sure you are happy with the time-lines specified.

CHAPTER FIVE

Practical issues – running the trial

Having thought through the scientific background to the proposed trial, having reviewed the protocol and had it approved by the ethics committee, having considered all the ethical implications of the trial, it is now necessary to face the cold day-to-day reality of conducting the study in your research unit, practice or hospital clinic. The scientific problem might be fascinating, but it is easy to lose sight of this in the mundane details of execution of the trial: scheduling patient visits, obtaining informed consent, checking entry criteria, collecting blood and urine samples, recording the data and filling in the forms correctly.

If you are serious about doing clinical research, you must organise yourself properly, allocating resources such as time, space, staff and training to the trials which you are conducting.

5.1   TIME

You must allocate enough time, not only to see the patients, but also to attend to the correct completion of documents, correspondence with the sponsor, dealing with data queries, meetings with monitors and your own staff, and generally managing the project locally. Clinical research cannot be effectively done with the left-overs of the working day, in the last quarter hour of the clinic or in the coffee breaks. It will help greatly if you can manage to appoint a study site coordinator (see below) to assume responsibility for most of the routine running of the project, but the research still requires a great deal of input of quality time from the investigator, who is ultimately responsible for the patients and the data. Try to allocate a sizeable portion of each day, or else a couple of dedicated and inviolable weekly sessions, to the research. It is fairly easy to plan the face-to-face time with patients; what few beginning investigators appreciate is the enormous amount of additional time that is required. It is probably wise to allocate up to two hours of non-contact work for every hour of patient contact in the project.

5.2　SPACE

You will also have to set aside substantial space for the project. Storage will be needed for the study drugs, which must be kept secure (locked) and well organised so that any given patient's supplies can be found easily, and so that an accurate track can be kept of what supplies remain at any given time. Shelf space will be needed for the case report forms, and perhaps your own set of notes; space will be needed for the investigator's site file, the investigator's brochure and the protocol; space will be needed for any additional equipment, for the kits in which you send blood and urine samples to the laboratory, and for storage of any samples which have to be kept locally (usually to send in a batch to the assay lab). In the long term you will have to think about archive space for storage of documents from completed trials: the GCP directives require retention of trial documents for 15 years. You may need a separate room in which to see the patients, or the study site coordinator may need a quiet room in which to work, telephone patients for appointments and carry out study-related procedures.

5.3　STAFFING

You will almost certainly have to allocate some staff to the conduct of the clinical trials. You may be fortunate enough to have access to the services of a research registrar, who should be utilised fully, bearing in mind that you have responsibilities towards him over training and supervision. Be careful that you allocate the registrar's time accurately according to the proportion of his salary that comes from the various sponsoring sources. Other personnel might include technicians, research nurses or a study site coordinator.

5.3.1　The study site coordinator

One of the most important people in the local team is the study site coordinator. Ideally this should be a nurse, or an experienced CRA (life science graduate). Recruit someone with relevant experience, or someone with common sense (preferably both) and send her on some appropriate courses or to conferences (for example ACRPI meetings), where she can meet others doing similar jobs, exchange ideas and find out what is going on in the world of clinical research.

Ideally the SSC should be a full-time position, with no routine clinical duties in the practice or ward, but if this is not feasible, ensure that she can at least devote a large proportion of her time to the research functions: do not expect her to do it in her spare time (even if you, as investigator, have to do the research in your spare time).

The main role of the SSC is to ensure the smooth day-to-day running of trials. She needs to pay attention to liaison and logistics; close liaison with practice managers or hospital administrators as well as the other clinical staff performing more routine functions. She will be the primary point of regular contact with the sponsor, liaising with CRAs over monitoring visits, receipt and dispatch of supplies, drugs, documents and samples. A major task will be the recruitment of suitable patients or volunteers, making their appointments to attend for study visits and follow-up, fitting in around the investigator's routine clinical work-load. She will be responsible for the study documentation, ensuring that the appropriate CRFs and patient notes are available for each visit, and are completed correctly and filed properly afterwards; she will attend to drug storage and supplies together with the associated record-keeping.

A large part of the task is checking everything – CRFs, patient logs, dispensing records and correspondence, and maintaining the investigator site file which the monitor should have provided. If any special equipment is used in the trial, its maintenance becomes her responsibility. She will have to deal with the processing of blood and urine samples (collecting, centrifuging, separating, freezing, storage), the labelling of bottles and records, and may find it useful to invent some forms or tables to help in the local management of records, samples, supplies and data. She might get involved in local procedures for data entry or processing. At a more managerial level, she might be responsible for writing some of the local standard operating procedures, and for training other local staff in their use, as well as in other aspects of clinical research and Good Clinical Practice. She might take responsibility for recruiting additional part-time or full-time research staff as required, and may have to spend a great deal of time gently nagging the investigator to do what is necessary to keep the trial going.

She may be able to assist the investigator in library work, conducting literature searches and obtaining copies of relevant publications. She will be the primary agent for damage limitation, recognising when things are going wrong and bringing them rapidly to the investigator's attention. She will possibly also keep the accounts relevant to the clinical trials work, ensuring that payment is received from the sponsor when the appropriate trial milestones are reached, submitting claims for expenses, filing tax returns and so on. Some of these functions require close liaison with the practice manager or hospital administrator.

Value your coordinator, and make sure that she feels valued – both financially and in the degree of trust and responsibility accorded (and by regular expressions of appreciation).

5.4   COMMUNICATION

Excellent communication is essential between all people involved in a clinical trial. You must of course maintain daily contact with your own staff, especially the study site coordinator, to receive updates on the progress of the subjects in the study, and regular scheduled local meetings are valuable to ensure that all issues are aired in a systematic way.

You must maintain regular contact with the sponsor's monitor; she will be paying periodic visits, but between visits you should keep in close touch. Try to allocate a regular weekly time to make contact, perhaps by telephone, but of course you must make additional contact as often as necessary in order to resolve issues that crop up along the way. It may be useful to devise a standardised format for routine progress reporting, so that a weekly or monthly summary of the state of recruitment can be sent.

Communication with the subjects is of course essential. They must be fully aware from the onset what is required of them, when they must visit, what restrictions on diet, alcohol or smoking apply, what concomitant drugs are allowed. They must know how to contact you in emergencies, or for reassurance, and must fully understand the need to report all adverse experiences and the taking of any medication.

Each time you see the subjects, the essential doctor–patient relationship must be maintained, and the subjects must not be made to feel they are simply 'guinea-pigs' in an experiment. I have witnessed relationships between investigators and subjects, particularly in trials on healthy volunteers, in which the subjects have been regarded almost as prisoners incarcerated in a concentration camp and made to conform to a regime of discipline and restriction that is wholly inappropriate; the attitude has been that 'we are paying them, so they should do what they are told'. A much more appropriate attitude is to regard the volunteers, whether healthy students or elderly patients, as our most valuable and essential asset in clinical research, who must be nurtured, cared for and treated with the greatest respect.

It is essential to keep careful records of all communication, so the primary advice is: WRITE EVERYTHING DOWN. Make a habit of taking notes of every telephone call, conversation or meeting and filing the note immediately.

5.4.1 Face-to-face conversations

Make a note immediately after any personal encounters or discussions about a trial, especially if decisions relevant to the conduct of the trial are taken. Place a copy of the note (signed and dated) in the study file or the subject's notes or both, and send a copy of the note to the other person if appropriate.

5.4.2 Telephone

Make sure you identify the person and position of anyone you speak to on the telephone. Try to identify the pertinent trial (in case you are involved in several) and which patient or subject is involved. Make a note of the conversation (it may help to have a pre-printed form) and place a signed dated copy in the relevant file. Send copies to anyone who needs to know; it may be helpful to send a letter to the other person confirming the contents of the telephone conversation.

5.4.3 Meetings

Make your own notes during meetings, recording particularly any decisions reached, any action points and any deadlines mentioned. Compare your notes with the official minutes when they arrive and discuss any discrepancies immediately. File a copy of your notes along with the official minutes.

5.4.4 Facsimile transmission and electronic mail

These are becoming more and more frequent as means of communication. While they can do much to speed the exchange of information, and often incorporate proof of date and time of transmission and receipt, be aware that some sponsors or their auditors do not find them acceptable as source documents for trials, and insist that proper original hard copies of relevant documents, transmitted by post or by hand, be stored in the study files.

5.4.5 Letters

File a copy of all your letters. Many auditors are nowadays no longer satisfied with the unsigned un-letterheaded 'carbon' copies of letters that traditionally get filed in hospital patient notes, but like to see a photocopy of the signed dated original that actually went out. ('How do I know that he signed it?') They sometimes even like to have someone sign to certify that this is a true and accurate photocopy!

5.5 TRAINING

There are two issues here: training for the investigator, and training for the support staff. In most trials, the sponsor or the responsible CRO will organise an investigators' meeting, just before or just after the beginning of the trial. Here, the organisers will present details of the drug, with background information on the therapeutic area, and some of the pre-clinical and clinical data underlying the design of the current trial. There will also be detailed discussions of the protocol, particularly regarding eligibility criteria and the strategy for recruitment of subjects, but also dwelling on measurement of the key outcome and safety variables, with instructions on how the CRF is to be completed and how drug supplies and blood samples are to be handled and stored.

While the investigator himself can gain a great deal from attendance at such a meeting, it is perhaps even more important that the study site coordinator or research nurse, who will be doing the bulk of the routine work, be enabled to attend, or at least that all the relevant information be passed on by the investigator. These meetings should not be regarded as 'perks' or junkets at the expense of the sponsor; in reality they are usually hard work, and although some sessions can be very long and appear rather dull, a lot of very important information is exchanged.

The investigator may undergo other forms of training either at his own or the sponsor's expense. Several of the national associations for clinical research or pharmaceutical physicians (such as BRAPP, ACRPI, AHPPI, the British Pharmacological Society and the Faculty of Pharmaceutical Medicine, as well as many societies for specialised branches of medicine) offer courses, symposia or meetings which may give valuable insights; many of these are recognised for continuing medical education (CME). Where possible, the ancillary staff must be encouraged to attend these as well as the investigator.

Unfortunately there is at present no recognised qualification for research nurses, who are largely left to their own devices to acquire the necessary skills. There is no officially specified training course, and until recently no forum where like-minded people could exchange information or discuss problems. Fortunately the ACRPI (an organisation largely catering for CRAs) has now started a group for investigator (or study) site coordinators, catering admirably for research nurses who should be actively encouraged to join.

Depending on the bias and interests of the investigator, and the therapeutic areas of involvement, the study site coordinators and research nurses could also be sent to courses and meetings on particular aspects of therapeutics or on general clinical pharmacology or simple statistical methods or whatever is appropriate. Be aware that all UK Registered Nurses are nowadays required to complete approved training on an ongoing basis (PREP – similar in concept to continuing medical education which is now becoming a requirement for doctors in many specialties), and it would be beneficial if some of the training could be relevant to clinical research. Try to get the sponsor to support such training, but even if funds are not forthcoming from that source, any money spent in training will be amply rewarded in terms of greater effectiveness of the research team.

All training activities should be documented. You should maintain a set of training records for yourself and all of your staff, and enter details of everything you do that is related to training. If you train your staff in lectures, seminars or discussion groups, enter it as training in your own record as well; teaching others is recognised as a valid form of training for yourself. Record all your attendances at postgraduate seminars, scientific meetings and conferences, all articles that you publish, and do the same for all the staff. Auditors and regulators are very keen to see a good complete set of training records, as evidence that you are serious about being an investigator and keeping yourself and your staff up to date, and it is only right that everyone at your site be given credit for all the training activities in which you are involved. A good set of records will also make it easier for you and your nurses to fulfil the requirements of PREP and CME.

5.6 DOCUMENTS

5.6.1 The investigator site file

The sponsor's monitor should supply each investigator with a file into which are placed all important documents relevant to a trial. This file should contain a signed copy of the protocol, the investigator's brochure, copies of ethics committee approval, forms to track the receipt and dispensing of trial medication, and many forms whose use one could not previously have imagined! If the monitor does not give you a file, create one yourself, to keep all relevant correspondence in one place, or better still nag the CRA until she supplies one. If you have already opened a file of your own, then transfer all the documents to the 'official' file once it has been supplied by the monitor. During the trial the monitor is supposed to check the investigator site file at regular intervals, and it is one of the first things that auditors inspect when they come to visit a site.

5.6.2 The investigator's brochure

The sponsor (or the CRO as agent) has a duty to supply the investigator with an investigator's brochure containing all the relevant information about the study drug, and the investigator has a duty to read it and become thoroughly familiar with its contents. It is in fact a great privilege to have access to this material, which should give insight into how the drug works and what trials have already been performed. There will be a great deal of information on the basic chemistry and pharmaceutical formulation: do not ignore this, because valuable clues to the mechanism of drug action may be found here, as well as an appreciation of potential problems of drug absorption, stability and shelf life. Pay particular attention to the toxicology, even if you find it rather dry and boring. (It has been said that if you find an excited toxicologist, you have a dead drug – in other words, the more routine and unexceptional the results of the toxicological trials, the better is the outlook for the drug and its developers.) Do not, however, allow yourself to be lulled into a false sense of security by the apparently bland reports – every so often a particularly significant finding will crop up which should alert the vigilant researcher about potential disasters or at least some important adverse reactions that might be expected.

5.6.3 The *curriculum vitae*

It is increasingly becoming a regulatory requirement that an investigator supply a current copy of his *curriculum vitae* to the sponsor; the CV is often attached to the investigator site file, and copies of CVs are attached to reports and sometimes even to protocols. The reasons are fairly obvious: auditors and regulators want to satisfy themselves that the people carrying out clinical research are properly qualified and experienced in the field relevant to the study, and adequately equipped to care for the patients on the trial in case of a medical emergency.

It is strongly advised that each investigator create and maintain a CV on file on a computer or word processor, to allow updated copies to be produced easily. It should be reviewed at regular intervals: of course every time one's employment or position changes, but also each time a paper is published or some new relevant experience is gained, each time training is undertaken or a course is attended.

The CV produced for placing in the investigator file is (or should be) different from the one used in applying for a job ('advertisement for myself') and should concentrate on listing qualifications, relevant posts and experience, additional relevant training, and a record of publications. It need not be longer than a couple of pages, and should be signed and dated by the investigator.

It is becoming usual for sponsors to ask for CVs of all the associates as well as the investigator: all the assistant doctors, even locum and on-call physicians, all the nursing, scientific and technical staff. The rule seems to be: if a person is likely to write in the CRF, a CV should be supplied. (It is, of course, also necessary to provide specimens of the signatures and initials of all persons writing in CRFs, to enable data entry staff to identify those authorised to make entries or corrections in the CRF.)

5.6.4 The clinical files (patient notes)

It is essential for any investigator conducting clinical research to keep excellent records. The patient records are invaluable, in fact essential as source documents for the monitor to verify. More important, they are your own permanent record of what happened, and of your patient's participation in a trial. If you work in a group practice or a hospital with a well-developed system of patient files, by all means use that system, provided you can guarantee ready access at all times. Otherwise you must develop your own system of notes and files, in which to write all relevant information about your trial subjects.

You are strongly advised to maintain a set of notes for *all* subjects, even healthy volunteers, so that you have a narrative record from trial to trial of each person's participation, and a note of any problems or adverse events experienced on previous trials. Try to keep a separate section in each patient's file for information relevant to each particular trial, if possible by using a cardboard file divider or a different colour of paper. The trial notes must contain a record of each visit (with the date), the purpose of the visit, and the essential events of that visit. In particular the signing of informed consent must be recorded, as well as the admission to a particular trial, and the randomization number or other subject identifier should be written in the patient's notes. All adverse events must be recorded, and this is an excellent place to include some narrative, particularly about severe or serious adverse events. If a monitor or sponsor subsequently requests further details, or more information than is normally given in the standard adverse event form, you have the data readily to hand together with any contemporaneous comments by attending physicians or nurses.

If you desire to keep your patient notes relevant to clinical trials on a computer instead of on paper, check with the sponsor's monitor about the acceptability of such records as source documents, and pay particular attention to details such as the provision of an audit trial if any corrections or amendments are made. Remember, too, the requirements of the Data Protection Act to inform the patient that his details are being stored on a computer.

Source data

You must write down the following source data in the patient notes or other clinical record, so that entries in the CRF can be verified:

Subject identity – name, address, date of birth, gender, ethnic origin.

Which trial the subject is trying to enter.

The fact that the investigator has given a written and oral explanation to the subject, and the fact that the subject has signed the consent form – include the date (as for *all* records).

Salient features of medical history and physical examination – discuss in advance with the monitor how detailed the description needs to be. Some are happy with 'Physical exam – NAD' ('nothing abnormal detected') while others require each body system to be described separately, with all positive and negative findings recorded.

Fulfilment of major entry criteria – diagnosis of target disease, if relevant.

State acceptability for trial; date of entry; dates of each visit, allocation of randomisation number and dispensing of drugs.

At visits after the initial screening, record the date of the visit, any adverse events and changes in or new concomitant medication, as well as confirming the continued use of study medication, or any non-compliance. This is also the place to record measurements of the primary study variable, if appropriate.

At the end of the trial, make an explicit entry stating that the subject has completed the trial (or withdrawn, or dropped out, as appropriate).

Resist the requests made by some monitors to make retrospective entries in the patient notes, copying or confirming data already collected in the CRF, so that there is a 'source document' for verification. At best this is silly; at worst, it can be fraudulent.

5.6.5 The case report form

This is the document in which all data about individual subjects or patients in a trial are recorded by the investigator and his staff. Insist on seeing the draft for the case report form early in the design phase and do not be afraid to comment on its content and layout; you and your staff are the ones who are going to use it, and it must be easy for you to use. It must be clear and unambiguous, and the entries should follow each other in logical progression. The time to make changes is *early* in the development, otherwise you run the risk of being stuck with an unmanageable document.

My own preference is to use a CRF in which the order of entries corresponds to the order in which procedures are performed and observations are made. It is very difficult, especially in a trial lasting a long time with many separate visits, to use a CRF in which all the blood pressure records are made on one page, all the blood samples are listed on another, and all the doses of drug are logged on a separate page. This may make life easy for data entry and data management staff, but can give rise to enormous numbers of errors and omissions at the point of data collection. If one considers the CRF as a series of 'bins' into which pieces of information have to be placed, it is always possible to rearrange the order of the bins once the data have been collected and placed into the computer; the important event is the placement of the data into the right bin by the person making the original observation, and this is made much easier if the CRF pages are arranged in a logical sequence. So the CRF must be designed primarily for the convenience of the recorder rather than the data managers. Perceptive data managers will recognise that if the recorder's task is made as easy as possible, the data manager's task will also be easier in the long run, because of the better quality of the data, with fewer errors and omissions.

Once the CRF design has been revised to your satisfaction, make sure that you and your staff become thoroughly familiar with its layout and contents. Know what you are expected to fill in, and do it completely and accurately. Use a black pen – monitors and auditors have a peculiar aversion to the use of any other colour, which probably stems from the days when only black ink could be reliably photocopied. Do not upset the monitors needlessly – throw away all your blue pens! Try to fill in every field of each page as you come to it. It takes only a few moments to fill in all the required information in a CRF at the time of patient contact; it is so much more tedious to be faced with a long list of omissions and corrections at the end.

In the long run, the only evidence of your part in the trial as an investigator will be the completed CRFs, so it is important that you get it right. Correctly completed CRFs, especially tidy ones, endear an investigator to the monitors and sponsors, who keep coming back to ask you to take part in more trials; poorly filled-in CRFs could ensure that this trial is your last.

5.6.6 Error correction

There are well-accepted, almost universal rules for the correction of errors in filling in CRFs and other clinical trial documents. As with all documents, we need to leave the record as clear, unambiguous and traceable as possible; it is unacceptable to obliterate the original record, for instance with correction fluid or by blacking-out or scribbling all over it. The proper way to make a correction is to strike through the mistaken entry with a single line, leaving it possible to read the original entry, and write the change as close to this as possible. The correction must be initialled and dated by the person making the alteration. Any attempt to alter data in any other way will incur the wrath of the monitor, the data entry clerk, the data manager, the auditor, the regulatory assessor and everyone else! It is essential that all staff working for an investigator are so familiar with these rules that they become second nature: if you teach your staff nothing else, teach them this.

5.6.7 Dealing with data queries

No matter how meticulous you are at filling in the CRF, there will be queries. Many will be raised by the monitor at routine site visits when she is checking through the latest batch of entries. Some monitors place a sticky 'Post-it' on the CRF page to signify the query, while others are expected to be more formal and submit a written list asking for changes. Do not get cross with the monitor; she has to ensure that all details are correct before she can 'lift' the CRF page and take it back to the office for data entry to proceed. CRAs are not themselves empowered to make any but the most minor changes to a CRF – the alterations must be made by the investigator or his staff, and the monitor will appreciate it if they can be made quickly. If you disagree with what is requested, it is better to discuss it openly than to become involved in a sequence of more and more acrimonious written com ments, though in the final analysis the investigator should retain the right and the ability to say 'don't be silly'.

Once the CRF pages have been taken back to the office (leaving a copy at the investigator site) the data entry clerks have to type the data into the computer database. They usually have little medical know-ledge and are only allowed to type what they see – they are not allowed to guess, correct the spelling, substitute words or otherwise modify the data. If something is illegible, they must raise a query and ask the investigator to clarify it. Once the data have been entered, they are subjected to validation checks and tests for plausibility; any values falling outside the data manager's pre-set ranges (for example for blood pres-sure) will be flagged, and the investigator will be asked to confirm them. So a systolic blood pressure which you have entered may well have actually been 240 mmHg, but it is almost certainly going to be queried; be prepared for it.

The raising of data queries does not imply criticism of the investigator, and he must not take them personally. Data entry clerks must obey the rules, so they must ask for clarification. Data managers have built validation checks into their systems to guard against errors, so they are obliged to ask for confirmation of unusual values. They are not imply-ing that you are wrong, they just want to make sure. The validity checks will also catch all sorts of errors; for example, it is very com-mon for an investigator in a hurry to enter today's date instead of a subject's date of birth, and the dates of events which follow each other are often reversed. Many data queries may seem trivial to you, but to data entry staff and many data managers all data have the same impor-tance and significance, so that it is just as important for a date or the contents of a [Yes/No] box to be correct as the result of a magnetic resonance imaging procedure. It is not the place of the data manage-ment staff to assign importance or weight to data, but to produce as complete and accurate a dataset as possible so that the statisticians, scientists and physicians can assess the trial's outcome and ascribe significance to the various items of information. Be patient with the data management staff, and they will be patient with you!

If you see the same data query coming again and again, check whether you or your staff are consistently making the same mistake, or whether you have misunderstood what is required. If you are sure of your own correctness, then talk to the data management staff or your monitor, for it is conceivable that their checking system is incorrect or flawed. Even data managers are fallible.

5.7   THE DRUGS – STORAGE AND CARE

The drugs are of course fundamental to the whole trial: without them there could be no trial. It is essential to get the delivery, storage and accountability of the drug right, so allocate sufficient dedicated space to store the study drugs, and sufficient time to check them on arrival, arrange them for convenient access, and keep the paperwork correctly filled in. Make sure that the drugs can be securely maintained under lock and key – the monitor will check this in advance and again during the study. Perform periodic checks of the number of dosage units in your possession: the monitor will do this as part of her duties at each visit, but it is preferable that you find out about any discrepancies before she does.

5.7.1   The randomisation code

In a randomised controlled trial, in which the investigator, the subject or both may be blinded as to which treatment is being given, the randomisation code is the primary determinant of treatment. It is usually constructed by a statistician, using tables of random numbers or a random algorithm on a computer. Treatment may be randomised over-all, when every subject has an exactly equal chance of being assigned any particular treatment, or may be randomised in blocks (such as groups of four or eight) or in a stratified manner (so that all young subjects form one group and all older subjects form another group). The drugs for the trial will be packed according to the randomisation code, so all the investigator usually has to do is to allocate the subject correctly to receive the next sequential treatment number and get the appropriate medication from the pre-packed boxes.

5.7.2 Breaking the code

The investigator in a double-blind trial is usually supplied with a set of sealed envelopes containing the key to break the code if it is necessary to find out what treatment a subject was receiving, for example if he develops a serious adverse experience which might require treatment with an antidote or other specific therapy. The code-break envelopes must be kept in a safe place which is nevertheless easy to find in an emergency, and must not be tampered with. The opening of a code-break envelope is regarded as an extremely significant occurrence in a clinical trial (almost more serious than a serious adverse event!) and anyone opening such an envelope must sign it and sign the CRF, giving reasons for opening the envelope. The facts must be communicated to the monitor as soon as possible after the event.

In most trials the code-break envelopes remain untouched, and are returned intact to the sponsor at the end of the trial (there should be a document to say this has happened).

5.8 HOW TO COPE WITH PROBLEMS OR DISASTERS

5.8.1 Adverse events (AEs)

We expect to record a certain number of adverse events (or adverse experiences) in every trial, and many of these will simply be intercurrent conditions or illnesses, or the chance non-specific ailments to which all flesh is heir. We must meticulously document all events, however, no matter how irrelevant they might seem, because someone who has access to the bigger picture, looking at the database of all adverse events in trials with that drug, might spot a connection, finding a cluster of unexplained symptoms that ring warning bells or suggest an alternative use for the drug. For example, someone may trip and sustain an injury on the way home from the clinic; this may seem irrelevant to the trial, but if enough people in different trials sustain accidental injuries, it might indicate some effect of the drug on balance, vigilance or alertness. This would need to be carefully examined, perhaps by initiating a separate trial including psychometric measurements. Or the chance finding of a high incidence of priapism among the volunteers on a trial of an anti-anginal drug might suggest the alternative use of the drug for the relief of impotence.

For most ordinary adverse events it is sufficient to make an entry in the patient's file and fill in an adverse event form, but if the event is in the least out of the ordinary, it is helpful to let the monitor know as soon as practicable. You should certainly draw the CRA's attention to it at the next regular monitoring visit. If the event is classifiable as a serious adverse event, it is of course mandatory to notify the monitor immediately.

5.8.2 Serious adverse events (SAEs)

A serious adverse event is defined by ICH as any event which is life-threatening or potentially life-threatening (all deaths are serious), causes hospitalisation or prolongation of existing hospitalisation, causes permanent injury or disability or is a congenital abnormality or birth defect. Many sponsors have their own definitions, which must include all these categories but might also introduce some others: some lists include any malignancy, some include pregnancy, and others include in the definition any withdrawal from the trial due to drug-related effects.

Whatever the precise definition, SAEs are a serious business. The most important thing is to report them early. In some countries the sponsor is required by law to report SAEs to the regulatory authority within 48 hours; there have been instances where the medical directors of large multinational pharmaceutical companies have been threatened with prison for failing to comply with all detailed regulations about filing SAE reports.

If the sponsor is to fulfil his responsibility for reporting, he obviously needs to get the information as quickly as possible. The investigator must, therefore, inform the sponsor as soon as the SAE becomes apparent. Telephone the monitor immediately; not the next morning, not the next working day, but right away, if necessary getting her out of bed. The protocol may say 'within 24 hours', but any delay reduces the time available to the sponsor for informing the authorities. Even if the event cannot remotely be connected with the trial drug (the bus in which the subject was riding spun off the road in icy weather) the clock starts ticking as soon as the investigator becomes aware of the event.

You cannot be content with sending the monitor a fax or leaving a message on a telephone answering machine or sending an e-mail message; you must be satisfied that the monitor has personally received the information, either by speaking to her directly or by receiving confirmation of receipt of a fax or e-mail. If the usual monitor is not available, the sponsor will have given an alternative contact telephone number, or a pager number, which must be used to contact someone responsible for dealing with the SAE. You must not rest until you have fulfilled your primary responsibility in this matter, of informing the sponsor of the occurrence of the SAE.

The monitor can then speedily initiate the next stage, by informing the licensing authority; again, the primary responsibility is to make the first contact, making the authority aware of the fact that a SAE has occurred. This first contact is the important one, and must occur within 48 hours of the event's coming to the notice of the investigator, for any trial involving the FDA (the time-lines vary with different licensing authorities).

Once the chain of notification has started, the details can be filled in at a later date, as more information becomes available. The details must, of course, be filled in, and very full records must be kept of all that happened, and of all contacts with the monitor and sponsor. The investigator also has a responsibility to inform the ethics committee of all serious adverse events, and copies of this notification must be filed with all the other correspondence in the investigator's site file.

5.8.3 Operational problems

Sometimes, despite the greatest of care, things go wrong during a clinical trial. A subject might be given the wrong dose of the drug, or a vital observation might be omitted; blood samples might be missed, collected late, mis-labelled or mixed up; the freezer for sample storage might break down so that samples thaw or are damaged; subjects might be admitted in violation of entry criteria, might transgress the restrictions on smoking, drugs or alcohol, or might withdraw or fail to turn up for no good reason at some critical stage of the trial; the recruitment targets might not be attained, either because of unrealistic optimism about the number of available subjects, or because of sheer bad luck; there may be grave errors or omissions in the completion of case report forms or other trial documents; the monitor may detect serious discrepancies in the stock of trial drugs or in the record-keeping.

In all cases, it is essential to maintain openness about the problem. Communicate with the sponsor's monitor as soon as possible. Talk to all staff involved in the trial. This is not the time to apportion blame: the person responsible for the error is usually already horribly upset and depressed about it and needs reassurance and persuasion not to resign on the spot. It is certainly not the time to attempt to cover up the mistake. The important thing it to ascertain facts: identify the problem fully, document it, find out why it happened, decide on curative action if it is possible, and take steps to ensure that it does not happen again.

Be reassured: when you first become aware of the error or disaster, it may seem as if the world, or at least your involvement in clinical research, has come to an abrupt and premature end. But on sober and careful reflection it will probably become apparent that all is not lost, that steps can be taken to limit the damage, that corrective action can be taken. Your problem is probably not the worst disaster that the sponsor has ever encountered, and there are probably even worse investigators around than you (though you must not take this as a licence to produce shoddy work at your centre). Be prepared to talk about the problem, with colleagues and other investigators, CRAs, the sponsor's medical staff. A solution can nearly always be found. Almost all your fellow investigators will recollect similar events in their own experience, and will reassure you that they have survived.

CHAPTER SIX

Publication

6.1 BY THE INVESTIGATOR

The investigator may wish to publish the results of the research because he feels the information is intrinsically interesting, needs to be communicated, or would enhance his (the investigator's) reputation and status. The sponsor, too, is often keen to have the data published, particularly if the results reflect favourably on his product. On the other hand, many sponsors are rather reticent about having trial results published. The issue of publication should be discussed thoroughly during the contract negotiation phase with the monitor or preferably someone more senior; if possible, get a written undertaking about when and where to publish, and who should write the paper. The protocol or contract often contains a bland statement about the desirability of publication, even though the sponsor may actually have no intention of publishing the report, and some more specific agreement should be in place before the trial starts.

On occasions the investigator wishes to publish, but the sponsor actively does not. This may be because the sponsor wishes to delay publication for commercial reasons (he does not want competitors to know of the success or failure of the treatment in a particular trial until the results of a whole sequence of trials are available) or because he does not want the particulars of an adverse reaction to be prematurely released. If the results of the trial are unfavourable to the sponsor's product, he may feel that publication is undesirable, and in fact may even try hard to block the publication despite the investigator's desire to publish. The investigator might feel that publication is in the public interest because of some previously unreported side effects or drug interactions, while the sponsor may feel that such news is likely to harm his product. There may be a purely commercial reason for a sponsor to wish to suppress publication, as in a recently reported case of a sponsor who for many years blocked publication of a report from a laboratory which had shown that low-cost generic thyroxine formulations were bioequivalent to a sponsor's higher-cost originator product.[13]

It is desirable to have extensive discussions between the interested parties in such cases, and try very hard to reach agreement about the strategy to be adopted, but if agreement cannot be reached and the investigator feels it is in the public interest for the data to be published, he must follow his conscience. He should always show the draft of any proposed paper to the sponsor and the other investigators, and preferably reach some sort of agreement over the text.

If you are unhappy with the sponsor's policy on publication, either before the trial or when the data are analysed, talk to the principal investigator and other investigators and try to formulate a joint approach, if necessary bringing combined pressure to bear on the sponsor to have the work published. It is most unfortunate if data are published against the wishes of the sponsor, but sometimes it has to be done, despite the potentially damaging consequences for the sponsor. It should be stressed to the sponsor that it is usually more damaging in the long term to be seen to have suppressed data than for the data to be published in the first place.

6.2   BY THE SPONSOR

On the other hand, the sponsor may encourage or even initiate publication of the research in the open literature in order to bring the product to the attention of the scientific and clinical (or perhaps commercial) community with a view to promoting the product. This can be a very favourable outcome for the investigator, especially if someone else can be persuaded to do the hard work of preparing the paper for publication.

The sponsor might be particularly keen to publish the results of a study if he feels that some real or apparent advantage over a competitor product has been demonstrated. Be very careful if you are asked to associate your name with such a publication. Insist that the sponsor be clearly identified as such: make sure he is not trying to pass off the paper as your 'independent' work showing that the sponsor's product is better than another. Read and check the text very carefully, making sure that there is no unfair slant, manipulation or suppression of the data in favour of the sponsor's product or to the detriment of the competitor.

Look closely at the periodical in which publication is intended: is it a peer-reviewed journal with a good reputation and high impact, or a 'pay-for-publication' un-refereed vehicle? Beware the symposium supplement to a journal, subsidised by the sponsor and rarely refereed: such publications may help inflate your *curriculum vitae*, but rarely enhance your reputation significantly. Try to suggest alternative target journals for your paper if you don't like the one suggested by the sponsor.

We are probably at the beginning of an explosion in electronic publication,[14] where papers can be placed on the Internet or World Wide Web and be read immediately by millions of computer users worldwide, but at present there seem to be few safeguards on the accuracy of such data, and refereeing or peer-review of papers in several such places is almost non-existent. Some of the more reputable journals have plans to include the comments of referees and also correspondence from the readers on the Internet site along with the original article, and this would make for a very exciting environment for publication, with almost instantaneous discussion and response from colleagues. Few clinical trial results have so far been published in this way, but it is likely that this route to publication will become more common within the next few years. Take extreme care that any such publication with which you are associated has the appropriate processes of checking and review attached to it.

6.3   THE INVESTIGATOR'S DUTY TO PUBLISH

It has been suggested that there is a duty to publish all the results of clinical research, that it is unethical to conduct a trial on human subjects without making the information available to the wider clinical community; thus a trial should not only be reported within the sponsor company or used for regulatory submission, but should be published in the open literature. Even trials with outcomes unfavourable to the sponsor or with negative or inconclusive results should be published, and this ought to ensure that people conducting meta-analyses over a number of clinical trials are able to obtain a fairer picture of the relative effectiveness of various treatments (at present most clinical trials which are published report only positive results). This suggestion begs the question of which journals are going to be prepared to publish negative findings or the results of boring routine trials performed merely for regulatory purposes: perhaps the Internet might in the future be a suitable repository for data which have no immediately arresting attraction for the editors of journals but nevertheless constitute useful information on the properties of drugs in development.

6.4   THE ISSUE OF AUTHORSHIP

Who should be included in the list of authors? Not all investigators are necessarily included, particularly in multi-centre multi-national trials, though the contribution of each participant in the trial should of course be acknowledged, perhaps in a list of investigators. As a guide, anyone who made a substantial contribution to the conception, design or realisation of the trial, to the analysis and interpretation of the data, or to the actual writing of the report, should be included as an author. Heads of department should not automatically be included in author lists of papers to which they have not made a material contribution. Several journals now publish clear guidelines defining the criteria for authorship, and emphasising the responsibility of each author for the content and data in the report.[15]

In the past, the person inside a pharmaceutical company's medical department who ultimately coordinated and wrote the clinical report was often not named as an author, but 'ghosted' the paper on behalf of one or more of the investigators. The reasons given were usually that the companies did not wish to be seen as sponsoring the research directly, but wanted the information to appear academically impeccable, looking as if it originated from the investigators. Recently most companies have allowed and even encouraged their staff members to be named as authors, thus enhancing the individuals' personal development and also adding to the companies' prestige by having members of staff with extensive lists of publications.

All authors of a published paper should have agreed to be named, all should have approved the text, and all should be prepared to defend the results and conclusions of the paper. Authorship is an enormous privilege, which carries with it a corresponding responsibility.

Postscript

I hope this book has succeeded in whetting the appetite of the potential clinical investigator, without causing undue anxiety about the enormous amount of paperwork and niggling administration involved. I have given pointers to means for coping with the myriad tasks associated with conducting a clinical trial.

I also hope it will provoke investigators to be prepared to say 'Don't be silly' when unreasonable demands are made of them. Scientific research is supposed to be exciting, intellectually stimulating and fulfilling to those engaged in it, and it would be a terrible shame if the trappings of excessive documentation and over-zealous checking were allowed to detract from this satisfaction.

Glossary and list of abbreviations

(This list refers largely to terms encountered in this book, but also contains other definitions which potential investigators may find useful.)

AA	Alcoholics Anonymous – a self-help group for people with drink problems
AA	Automobile Association – a vehicle rescue service and motorists' pressure group
ABPI	Association of the British Pharmaceutical Industry
ACE	Angiotensin Converting Enzyme. Responsible for activating an inert protein in plasma, making it into a potent vasoconstrictor. ACE inhibitors block this effect, and are widely used as antihypertensives
ACLS	Advanced Cardiac Life Support – resuscitation
ACRPI	Association of Clinical Research for the Pharmaceutical Industry (the professional body for CRAs)
AE	Adverse Event (or Adverse Experience)
AF	Atrial Fibrillation
AHPPI	Association for Human Pharmacology in the Pharmaceutical Industry
AICRC	Association of Independent Clinical Research Contractors
AIDS	Acquired Immune Deficiency Syndrome (in French, SIDA)
ANDA	Abbreviated New Drug Application (see NDA). Application to FDA for approval to market generic drugs
ARSAC	Administration of Radioactive Substances Advisory Committee (United Kingdom). Body from whom

approval must be sought before undertaking radio-label studies in humans

AUC   Area under the concentration/time curve; usually applied to data on plasma or urine concentrations of drugs. May be subscripted to indicate the interval over which integration is performed, e.g. $AUC_{0-\infty}$ or $AUC[24-48h]$

BA   Bachelor of Arts – awarded as the primary degree, sometimes even for science subjects (especially at Oxford and Cambridge and the Open University), but more usually for non-scientific subjects

BMA   British Medical Association.

BMJ   *British Medical Journal* – published by the BMA

BNF   British National Formulary

BP   Blood Pressure

BP   British Pharmacopoeia

BPC   British Pharmacopoeia Codex

BPS   British Pharmacological Society

BRAPP   British Association of Pharmaceutical Physicians (formerly AMAPI – Association of Medical Advisors in the Pharmaceutical Industry)

BSc   Bachelor of Science – the most usual primary qualification in science at European and US universities

CABG   Coronary Artery Bypass Graft operation (pronounced CABBAGE)

CD-ROM   Compact Disk Read-Only Memory: a high-density medium based on the compact disk laser optical system originally designed for music systems, now used for storage of computer information

CEO   Chief Executive Officer

CME   Continuing Medical Education

COSTART   Coding Symbols for a Thesaurus of Adverse Reaction Terms

CPMP   Committee for Proprietary Medicinal Products (European Union)

CRA   Clinical Research Associate – an employee of a pharmaceutical sponsor company or a CRO, usually a life science graduate, a nurse or a physician, who undertakes monitoring and related tasks

CRF   Case Record Form (or Clinical Report Form) – the document into which all details about an individual

	subject in a clinical trial are to be entered, including all measurements and observations
CRO	Contract Research Organisation – a company offering facilities for organising, conducting, monitoring, analysing and reporting pre-clinical or clinical pharmaceutical research on behalf of a sponsor, on a commercial basis
CSM	Committee on Safety of Medicines (United Kingdom)
CTC	Clinical Trial Certificate (United Kingdom – authority from CSM to conduct a trial)
CTMP	Certificate for a Clinical Trial on a Marketed Product (United Kingdom)
CTX	Clinical Trial Certificate Exemption (United Kingdom – authority to conduct a trial, obtained from MCA without submitting a full dossier to CSM)
CV	*Curriculum Vitae*
CVA	Cerebrovascular Accident – a stroke or apoplexy usually due to cerebral thrombosis or cerebral haemorrhage
CVCP	Committee of Vice-Chancellors and Principals (of United Kingdom Universities)
DDX	Doctor's and Dentist's Clinical Trial Certificate Exemption (United Kingdom) – authority for an individual investigator to initiate and undertake a piece of unsponsored (or self-sponsored) clinical research
Dip Pharm Med	Diploma in Pharmaceutical Medicine (of the Royal College of Physicians)
DNA	Deoxyribonucleic acid (in genetics and molecular biology)
DNA	Did Not Appear (in hospital notes – 'no show')
DOS	Disk Operating System (in computers), especially MS-DOS, MicroSoft DOS. The program that keeps the computer running, and launches all of the other application programs
DSc	Doctor of Science – a degree awarded in recognition of a substantial contribution to research, usually over several years or even decades. A large number of published papers are usually bound together and submitted as a dissertation
EC	European Community

ECG	Electrocardiograph, electrocardiogram (also EKG – particularly in US)
EEG	Electroencephalograph, electroencephalogram
ELISA	Enzyme-linked immunosorbent assay – a standard laboratory method to measure concentrations of many substances in body fluids
E-mail	Electronic mail – a technique making use of computer networks, especially the Internet, for sending messages or documents to other users of the network. Usually a very rapid method of communication – enthusiasts refer to the conventional postal system as 'snail mail'
EMEA	European Medicines Evaluation Agency (European Union)
EU	European Union
EuP	European Pharmacopoeia
FASEB	Federation of American Societies for Experimental Biology
FDA	Food and Drug Administration (United States) – the main US regulatory body for pharmaceuticals
FRCA	Fellow of the Royal College of Anaesthetists
FRCR	Fellow of the Royal College of Radiologists
FRCS	Fellow of the Royal College of Surgeons
FRS	Fellow of the Royal Society – an extremely prestigious award made in recognition of outstanding scientific contributions
GC, GC/MS	Gas Chromatography, without or with Mass Spectroscopy
GCP	Good Clinical (Research) Practice
GLP	Good Laboratory Practice
GMC	General Medical Council (United Kingdom). Maintains official register of qualificd doctors
GMP	Good Manufacturing Practice
GP	General Practitioner, primary care physician, family practitioner.
HIV	Human Immunodeficiency Virus
HMSO	Her Majesty's Stationery Office. The UK government publisher
HNC, HND	Higher National Certificate or Diploma. Non-university award for completion of technical training; standard may be at least equivalent to pass degree level. HNC is for part-time courses, HND full-time

HPLC	High Pressure (or Performance) Liquid Chromatography – a standard bioanalytical technique
HV	Health Visitor – a health worker, basically trained as a nurse, who has a role in the community, chiefly in preventive medicine
HV	Healthy Volunteer (in Phase I studies)
IBM	International Business Machines – a major manufacturer of computers. Especially used in IBM-PC (see PC)
ICH	International Conference on Harmonisation of technical requirements for registration of pharmaceuticals for human use (members from US, EC, Japan)
IDDM	Insulin-dependent diabetes mellitus, i.e. usually juvenile onset or Type I diabetes
IFAPP	International Federation of Associations of Pharmaceutical Physicians
IM or i.m.	Intramuscular (injection)
IND	Investigational New Drug (US) – an application is filed with the FDA for authority to conduct clinical trials
IP or i.p.	Intraperitoneal (injection)
IRB	Institutional Review Board (US – equivalent to Local Research Ethics Committee)
IT	Information Technology (a pretentious term for computer science)
IV or i.v.	Intravenous (injection or infusion)
JAMA	*Journal of the American Medical Association*
kcal	Kilocalorie (one thousand calories). A unit of heat or energy: one calorie is the energy required to raise the temperature of 1 cm^3 of water at $0\,^\circ C$ by $1\,^\circ C$. The calorie and kilocalorie are widely used as units in nutrition, but are non-SI units. It is more correct to specify the energy value of foods in kiloJoules or MegaJoules, the proper SI Units
kJ, MJ	KiloJoule, MegaJoule. The SI unit of energy is the Joule, which should be used in nutritional studies. One kilocalorie = 4.18 kJ
LRCP, MRCS	Licentiate of the Royal College of Physicians and Member of the Royal College of Surgeons – the Conjoint Diploma of basic qualification in medicine awarded by the London Colleges, often to doctors qualifying without a university degree

LREC	Local Research Ethics Committee
MA	Master of Arts – a postgraduate qualification granted by many universities in recognition of additional courses of study undertaken after the primary degree. Often given even if the primary degree was in science or medicine (especially at Oxford and Cambridge)
MAO	Monoamine Oxidase. An enzyme which breaks down substances in the adrenaline family. MAO inhibitors are used in psychiatry as antidepressants, but may interact with many cardiovascular drugs
MB	Bachelor of Medicine (sometimes BM) – the primary medical qualification in British universities. Usually granted along with BS or ChB or BCh – Bachelor of Surgery, sometimes also with BAO – Bachelor of (the Art of) Obstetrics
MCA	Medicines Control Agency (United Kingdom)
MD	Doctor of Medicine (sometimes DM) – in Europe, a higher research degree awarded after submission of a dissertation or thesis to the university which granted the primary medical qualification. In North America the MD is the primary medical qualification, but has the status of a postgraduate degree because all medical students obtain a primary bachelor's degree (e.g. BSc, BA) before entering medical school
MD	Managing Director, Medical Director
MFPM	Member of the Faculty of Pharmaceutical Medicine (of the Royal Colleges of Physicians). Also AFPM (Associate) and FFPM (Fellow)
MI	Myocardial Infarct(ion) – or Coronary Thrombosis (CT). Also Mitral Incompetence
MLSO	Medical Laboratory Scientific Officer
mmHg	Millimetre of Mercury – empirical measure of pressure (especially arterial blood pressure) which has withstood all attempts to replace it by the SI unit, the pascal or kilopascal
MPhil	Master of Philosophy – a degree awarded in recognition of a dissertation describing research work of a standard or scope rather lower than that which would qualify for a Doctorate
MRC	Medical Research Council (United Kingdom, Canada, Australia). A major grant-giving body

MRCOG	Member of the Royal College of Obstetricians and Gynaecologists. Also FRCOG (Fellow)
MRCP	Member of the Royal College of Physicians. Also FRCP (Fellow)
MREC	Multi-Centre Research Ethics Committee
MRPS	Member of the Royal Pharmaceutical Society. Denotes registered pharmacist. Also FRPS (Fellow). Formerly MPS, FPS. The Society maintains the official register of pharmacists
MSc	Master of Science – postgraduate degree, often given at the end of a prescribed course of higher scientific training, but sometimes also requiring a short dissertation.
NAD	Nothing Abnormal Detected – often written in clinical notes
NATO	North Atlantic Treaty Organization (in French, OTAN)
NDA	New Drug Application (US) – an application to the FDA for marketing authorisation for a new chemical entity. Equivalent to Product Licence Application in EU
NIDDM	Non-insulin dependent diabetes mellitus – i.e. usually maturity onset or Type II diabetes
NHS	National Health Service (in UK)
NOAEL	No Adverse Effect Level: dose of a drug which is just below the threshold at which toxicity is detected (or the highest dose at which there are no toxic effects)
NSAID	Non Steroidal Anti-Inflammatory Drug
OTC	Over-the-counter, i.e. a drug or appliance available without prescription. (See, by contrast, POM)
PC	Personal Computer
PD	Pharmacodynamics – the study of the effects of a drug on its target organ
pH	The negative logarithm of the hydrogen ion concentration in a solution – an index of acidity or alkalinity. Solutions with pH less than 7 are acid, those above 7 are alkaline
PhD	Doctor of Philosophy (also DPhil) – postgraduate degree awarded in recognition of a substantial piece of research work submitted as a dissertation or thesis (in almost any discipline). May also (especially in North America) require the completion of specified

	course-work, sometimes leading to an MSc as an intermediate stage. (*Philosophy* in its widest sense – love of thought – includes natural philosophy)
PK	Pharmacokinetics – the study of the Absorption, Distribution, Metabolism and Elimination (ADME) of a drug in the body
PK/PD	Pharmacokinetic/Pharmacodynamic interaction: a study of the extent to which plasma or tissue concentrations of drugs directly affect the action measured in the target organ
pK, pKa	The negative logarithm of the dissociation constant of an ionic species in solution
PO or p.o.	Per Os (i.e. Oral)
POM	Prescription-only medicine: available only on prescription by a doctor or dentist. (Compare OTC)
PR or p.r.	*Per rectum* (rectal examination, or administration of drugs)
PR interval	On ECG, the interval between the onset of atrial depolarisation and ventricular depolarisation
PREP	Post-Registration Education and Practice (for UK Registered Nurses and midwives). A minimum of five study days over three years
PRN	*Pro re nata*, as required (especially of drug dosage)
PV or p.v.	*Per vaginem* (vaginal examination, or administration of drugs)
QA	Quality Assurance – a check that systems to ensure the correct conduct of clinical trials are in place and are being implemented
QC	Quality Control – the systematic check of individual items of data, procedures, documents and activities during a process or trial
RAC	Royal Automobile Club – vehicle recovery service and motorists' pressure group
RAM	Random Access Memory – Read/Write memory for computers
RBC	Red Blood Cells
RCN, RCM	Royal College of Nurses, Midwives. Professional bodies which aim to set high standards and maintain the professional position of nurses and midwives, but do not grant degrees or diplomas
RGN	Registered General Nurse – formerly SRN, State Registered Nurse

RIA	Radio immunoassay – a standard laboratory method for measuring many substances in body fluids
RN	Registered Nurse (US). (Also Royal Navy)
ROM	Read-Only Memory: computer memory, usually containing programs or other information which cannot or need not be changed
RSM	Royal Society of Medicine (London)
SAE	Serious Adverse Event (or Experience) – one which requires immediate reporting to sponsor, to regulatory authorities and to Ethics Committee. Usually defined as being fatal or life-threatening, causing permanent disability, requiring hospitalization or involving cancer, congenital defect or overdose
SAE	Stamped, Addressed Envelope (or reply-paid envelope) to encourage recipients of correspondence to respond
SAS	Statistical Analysis System – software produced by SAS Inc., widely used for analysis of clinical trials
SC or s.c.	Subcutaneous (injection)
SDV	Source Document (or Data) Verification – the process of verifying each entry in a Case Record Form against some Source Document such as the patient's hospital notes
SI	*Système Internationale* – a coherent system for defining, naming and abbreviating scientific units in physics, chemistry and biology
SOP	Standard Operating Procedure
SQL	Structured Query Language – used to interrogate computer databases (pronounced SEQUEL)
SVT	Supraventricular (usually atrial) tachycardia
TIA	Transient Ischaemic Attack (usually refers to *cerebral* ischaemia)
UK	United Kingdom (of Great Britain and Northern Ireland)
UKCC	United Kingdom Central Committee for Nurses, Midwives and Health Visitors (maintains official registers)
UN	United Nations
UNESCO	United Nations Educational, Scientific and Cultural Organization
UPS	Uninterruptible Power Supply – back-up power supply for computers and other electronic equipment in event of mains power failure

US (A)	United States (of America)
USP	United States Pharmacopoeia
UV	Ultraviolet
VF	Ventricular Fibrillation
VT	Ventricular Tachycardia
WBC	White Blood Cells
WHO	World Health Organization
WHO-ART	WHO dictionary of Adverse Reaction Terms (an alternative to COSTART)

Notes

1. D. Luscombe and P.D. Stonier (eds), *Clinical Research Manual* (Haslemere: Euromed Communications, 1994); J.P. Griffin, J. O'Grady and F.O. Wells, *The Textbook of Pharmaceutical Medicine* (Belfast: Queen's University, 1993).
2. *Directory of Grant-Making Trusts*, 13th Edition (Tonbridge: Charities Aid Foundation 1993).
3. P.B. Medawar, *Advice to a Young Scientist* (London: Pan Books, 1979), pp. 45–8.
4. *Recommendations Guiding Physicians in Biomedical Research Involving Human Subjects*. Adopted by the 18th World Medical Assembly, Helsinki, Finland, June 1964 and amended by the 29th World Medical Assembly, Tokyo, Japan, October 1975, 35th World Assembly, Venice, Italy, October 1983, 41st World Medical Assembly, Hong Kong, September 1989, and the 48th General Assembly, Somerset West, Republic of South Africa, October 1996.
5. W.G. McBride, 'Thalidomide and congenital abnormalities', *British Medical Journal* **5320**, 1962, p. 1681.
6. 'Guidelines for good clinical practice', *The Rules Governing Medicinal Products in the European Community*, Vol. III (Addendum), July 1990; Directive 91/507/EEC, Commission of the European Communities.
7. 'Federal policy for the protection of human subjects: notices and rules', *Federal Register* **56**(117), 18 June 1991, pp. 28003–32; 'Obligations of sponsors and monitors of clinical investigations: proposed rules', *Federal Register* **42**, 27 September 1977, pp. 49621–6.
8. *ICH Harmonised Tripartite Guideline for Good Clinical Practice* (Geneva: ICH Secretariat, 1996).

9. *Guidelines on Good Clinical Research Practice* (London: The Association of the British Pharmaceutical Industry, 1988).

10. R. Smith, 'The need for a national body on research misconduct', *British Medical Journal* **316**, 1998, pp. 1686–7. Also several other articles in the same issue of the *BMJ*.

11. Data Protection Act 1984 (London: Her Majesty's Stationery Office).

12. *Guidelines. Clinical Trials – Compensation for Medicine-Induced Injury* (London: The Association of the British Pharmaceutical Industry, 1983); *Guidelines for Medical Experiments in Non-Patient Human Volunteers* (London: The Association of the British Pharmaceutical Industry, 1988).

13. J. Wise, 'Research suppressed for seven years by drug company', *British Medical Journal* **314**, 1997, p. 1145. Citing *Journal of the American Medical Association* **277**, 1997, pp. 1205–18.

14. L. Bero, 'The electronic future: what might an online scientific paper look like in five years' time?', *British Medical Journal* **315**, 1997, p. 1692.

15. 'Uniform requirements for manuscripts submitted to biomedical journals', *New England Journal of Medicine* **336**, 1997, pp. 309–15.

Index

adverse events 51
  serious 18–19, 35, 52
archive 38
audit 12, 22, 27, 46
authorship 58

biologist 8
biology 7

case report form *see* CRF
chemistry 7, 44
client/server 2
clinical files 45
clinical pharmacologist 1
communication 40
compensation 30, 33, 35
confidentiality 31
consent 14, 18, 20, 27, 31
consent form 20–1, 46
CME 43
contract 16, 28, 55
  research *see* CRO
CRF 27, 31–3, 42, 46–51
CRO 1, 3, 4, 22, 28
CTX 19
curiosity-driven 3
curriculum vitae 45

data entry 39, 48–9
data managers 25, 47–9
Data Protection Act 31, 46
data queries 26, 37, 48
DDX 3
Declaration of Helsinki 5, 13

drug
  development 7
  registration 10
  storage 50

eligibility criteria 34, 42
error correction 48
ethics committee 20, 35, 53
  local (LREC) 14
  multi-centre (MREC) 14
European Union 11

FDA 11, 12, 53
fraud 12, 17

GCP 11, 27, 32, 39
general practitioner 1
generic 7, 56

ICH 11, 13, 23
Institutional Review Board 15
insurance 30, 33
internet 57
investigator
  brochure 30, 38, 44
  duties 17, 30
  grant 16, 19, 28
  principal 18, 33
  site file 18, 38–9, 44, 53
investigators' meeting 19, 42

LD_{50} 8

marketing
  authorisation 7
  licence 10